SpringerBriefs in Psychology

Advances in Child and Family Policy and Practice

SpringerBriefs present concise summaries of cutting-edge research and practical applications across a wide spectrum of fields. Featuring compact volumes of 50 to 125 pages, the series covers a range of content from professional to academic. Typical topics might include:

- A timely report of state-of-the-art analytical techniques
- A bridge between new research results as published in journal articles and a contextual literature review
- A snapshot of a hot or emerging topic
- An in-depth case study or clinical example
- A presentation of core concepts that readers must understand to make independent contributions

SpringerBriefs in Psychology showcase emerging theory, empirical research, and practical application in a wide variety of topics in psychology and related fields. Briefs are characterized by fast, global electronic dissemination, standard publishing contracts, standardized manuscript preparation and formatting guidelines, and expedited production schedules.

More information about this series at https://link.springer.com/bookseries/10143

Series Editor
Lisa A. Gennetian, Duke Sanford School of Public Policy
Duke University
Durham, North Carolina, USA
Advances in Child and Family Policy and Practice is a SpringerBriefs in Psychology Series published in collaboration with the Society for Child and Family Policy and Practice (Division 37 of the American Psychological Association). The series serves as a forum for the scholarly review of psychological knowledge relevant to social issues, public policy, and service delivery that affects child and family development.

Briefs are comprehensive reviews of contemporary issues in the lives of children, youth, and families living in a society that values diversity, equity, and inclusion. Briefs examine a social, policy, systemic, service delivery, family, or developmental issue relevant to the well-being of children from birth through emerging adulthood. Briefs may also focus on professional, legal, and ethical issues that affect the structure and delivery of social, educational, and healthcare services to children, youth, and families.

Briefs may be a monograph written by a single author or several authors; they may also be an integrated set of briefer papers that explore different dimensions of a specific topic organized by a guest editor or editors. They may be proposed by a lead author or guest editor, and they may be solicited by the editorial board. Collections of original research reports are not considered for publication. All submissions are peer reviewed to ensure they represent a substantive contribution to the literature on child and family policy and practice. Each brief must also include a summary for use in education and advocacy.

John P. Ackerman • Lisa M. Horowitz
Editors

Youth Suicide Prevention and Intervention

Best Practices and Policy Implications

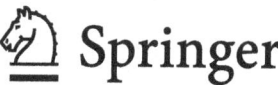 Springer

Editors
John P. Ackerman
Center for Suicide Prevention and Research
Nationwide Children's Hospital
Columbus, OH, USA

Lisa M. Horowitz
National Institute of Mental Health,
Intramural Research Program, National
Institutes of Health
Bethesda, MD, USA

ISSN 2192-8363   ISSN 2192-8371   (electronic)
SpringerBriefs in Psychology
ISBN 978-3-031-06126-4   ISBN 978-3-031-06127-1   (eBook)
https://doi.org/10.1007/978-3-031-06127-1

This Springer imprint is published by the registered company Springer Nature Switzerland AG
The registered company address is: Gewerbestrasse 11, 6330 Cham, Switzerland

May the sobering statistics, past and present, and the tragic death of every single youth who has died by suicide be a call to action. This book is dedicated to the caring adults who seek to better understand and support youth at risk for suicide – may you be empowered to uncover answers that lead to better interventions and systems of care; may you initiate critical conversations and provide compassionate support when it is needed; and may you take every opportunity to foster resilience and help youth navigate life's challenges so that more lives can be saved. This book is also dedicated to suicide attempt survivors, suicide loss survivors, and all those impacted by suicidal thoughts and behaviors. Your experiences and your voices guide our work. We hope that these chapters contribute to a better understanding of suicide for readers and encourage policies that advance innovative and effective suicide prevention efforts in all communities.

Preface

Suicide among youth in the USA has been, and continues to be, a public health crisis. Tragically, there have been persistent increases in youth suicide rates in recent years despite increased resources and effort directed at this problem. This is not to suggest that important work is not being done. Quite the opposite is true. As you will see throughout this volume, our knowledge of factors that place young people at risk for suicide is increasing, and our ability to identify, assess, and treat youth at imminent risk is improving. Additionally, understanding the wide array of cultural contexts that dynamically influence risk and protective factors drives a pressing need for more research and interventions that are more culturally applicable to understudied and underserved populations that may be at highest risk. Despite these advances, there are many gaps in what we know about youth suicide and how that is communicated to the public, disseminated in our communities, and translated into effective reduction of suicide and suicidal behavior.

The goal of this volume is to provide clinicians, researchers, policy makers, or anyone passionate about suicide prevention research with current information across key domains of youth suicide prevention in a digestible format. The chapters included in this volume are not intended to provide an all-encompassing examination of respective topics; rather, authors summarize current research, identify existing gaps in science and practice, and provide recommendations for future research, training, practice, and policy. This format was chosen intentionally so that individuals could pick a topic and quickly understand what subject matter experts in that field deem to be the most pressing issues with perspective on how to meaningfully advance youth suicide prevention efforts.

Chapters in this volume are grouped according to similar interests, and readers may choose to focus on chapters of specific sections. Nevertheless, we encourage readers to spend time with all the chapters, as each offers unique insight to advancing youth suicide prevention and policy efforts. While there is much progress yet to be made, years of research have built a foundation which can serve as a roadmap moving forward. Topics addressed in this volume include:

- Foundations of youth suicide prevention
- Suicide prevention and postvention in school settings
- Suicide-specific interventions
- Cultural considerations and specific populations
- Improving quality of suicide care across systems
- Incorporating lived experience perspective into research and practice

This series addresses a large range of topics; however, due to limited space, it is not inclusive of all the current efforts in suicide prevention. While not included in this series, we encourage readers to also inform themselves of other noteworthy suicide prevention efforts, such as social media campaigns and other preventative treatment options. We would also like to call attention to the Blueprint for Youth Suicide Prevention, located on the American Academy of Pediatrics website (www. aap.org/suicideprevention).

At times, the challenges of reducing suicide may seem insurmountable. Yet, the sobering statistics of youth suicide amplify the continued need for a call to action. It is our belief that the chapters in this volume, drawing from the wisdom and experience of some of the country's leading suicide prevention experts and voices of lived experience, provide guidance on how we can continue to improve prevention efforts and save lives. Our hope is that this volume accelerates the pace of youth suicide prevention efforts and encourages readers to embrace their role in suicide prevention. Every one of us can make a difference.

Columbus, OH, USA   John P. Ackerman
Bethesda, MD, USA   Lisa M. Horowitz

Acknowledgements

We would like to thank Nathan J. Lowry, Patrick C. Ryan, and Annabelle M. Mournet for their incredible dedication and assistance in the publication of this Advance Volume.

A special thank you to the Nationwide Children's Hospital Foundation and Big Lots Behavioral Health Services for making this Advance Volume open access and publicly available without cost. To ensure that suicide prevention is equitable, we felt that the information contained in this volume needed to be accessible to all partners. We appreciate Nationwide Children's Hospital for supporting this vision. This Advance Volume was also supported in part by the Intramural Research Program of the National Institute of Mental Health, National Institutes of Health (Annual Report Number ZIAMH002922).

Contents

Contributors

Seth Abrutyn Department of Sociology, University of British Columbia, Vancouver, BC, Canada

John P. Ackerman Big Lots Behavioral Health Services, Nationwide Children's Hospital, Columbus, OH, USA

Department Psychiatry & Behavioral Health, The Ohio State University College of Medicine, Columbus, OH, USA

Bart Andrews Behavioral Health Response (BHR), St. Louis, MO, USA

Joan Asarnow Department of Psychiatry and Biobehavioral Sciences, University of California, Los Angeles, CA, USA

Lynsay Ayer RAND Corporation, Santa Monica, CA, USA

Elizabeth D. Ballard Section on the Neurobiology and Treatment of Mood Disorders, National Institute of Mental Health, Bethesda, MD, USA

Samanta Boddapati Big Lots Behavioral Health Services, Nationwide Children's Hospital, Columbus, OH, USA

Department Psychiatry & Behavioral Health, The Ohio State University College of Medicine, Columbus, OH, USA

Mandy Bowlin Behavioral Health Response (BHR), St. Louis, MO, USA

Rhonda C. Boyd Department of Child and Adolescent Psychiatry and Behavioral Sciences at the Children's Hospital of Philadelphia and the University of Pennsylvania Perelman School of Medicine, Philadelphia, PA, USA

Jeffrey A. Bridge Center for Suicide Prevention and Research, Abigail Wexner Research Institute at Nationwide Children's Hospital, Columbus, OH, USA

Departments of Pediatrics, Psychiatry & Behavioral Health, The Ohio State University College of Medicine, Columbus, OH, USA

Teresa Brockie Johns Hopkins School of Nursing, Baltimore, MD, USA

John V. Campo Johns Hopkins School of Medicine, Baltimore, MD, USA

Julie Cerel University of Kentucky, College of Social Work, Lexington, KY, USA

Meredith R. Chapman Big Lots Behavioral Health Services, Nationwide Children's Hospital, Columbus, OH, USA

Department of Psychiatry & Behavioral Health, The Ohio State University College of Medicine, Columbus, OH, USA

Joyce Chu Palo Alto University, Palo Alto, CA, USA

Laura Coleman Behavioral Health Response (BHR), St. Louis, MO, USA

Catherine Cox Behavioral Health Response (BHR), St. Louis, MO, USA

Mary F. Cwik Johns Hopkins Bloomberg School of Public Health, Baltimore, MD, USA

Johns Hopkins School of Medicine, Baltimore, MD, USA

Walter Dempsey Department of Biostatistics, University of Michigan, Ann Arbor, MI, USA

Sarah Diefendorf Department of Sociology, Indiana University Bloomington, Bloomington, IN, USA

Sarah M. Edwards University of Maryland School of Medicine, Baltimore, MD, USA

Amanda Fox Community Crisis Services, Inc., Hyattsville, MD, USA

Kathryn R. Fox Department of Psychology, University of Denver, Denver, CO, USA

Julie Goldstein Grumet Zero Suicide Institute, Education Development Center, Waltham, MA, USA

Jane Hamel-Lambert Nationwide Children's Hospital, Columbus, OH, USA

The Ohio State University, Columbus, OH, USA

Sharon Hoover National Center for School Mental Health, University of Maryland, MD, USA

Lisa M. Horowitz National Institute of Mental Health, Bethesda, Maryland, USA

Katie Johanning-Gray Nationwide Children's Hospital, Columbus, OH, USA

The Ohio State University, Columbus, OH, USA

Oula Khoury Big Lots Behavioral Health Services, Nationwide Children's Hospital, Columbus, OH, USA

Department of Pediatrics, The Ohio State University College of Medicine, Columbus, OH, USA

Palo Alto University, Palo Alto, CA, USA

Tamar Kodish Department of Psychiatry and Biobehavioral Sciences, University of California, Los Angeles, CA, USA

W. Cole Lawson Department of Psychology, University of Denver, Denver, CO, USA

Nathan J. Lowry National Institute of Mental Health, Bethesda, Maryland, USA

Kurt D. Michael Appalachian State University, Boone, NC, USA

Maureen F. Monahan New York State Psychiatric Institute, New York, NY, USA

Department of Psychiatry, Columbia University Irving Medical Center, New York, NY, USA

Annabelle M. Mournet National Institute of Mental Health, Bethesda, Maryland, USA

Anna Mueller Department of Sociology, Indiana University Bloomington, Bloomington, IN, USA

Juliana F. Ng Palo Alto University, Palo Alto, CA, USA

Kerri Nickerson American Institutes for Research, Arlington, VA, USA

Matthew K. Nock Department of Psychology, Harvard University, Cambridge, MA, USA

Sam E. O'Neill Palo Alto University, Palo Alto, CA, USA

Maryland Pao Office of the Clinical Director, National Institute of Mental Health, National Institutes of Health, Bethesda, MD, USA

Ujjwal Ramtekkar University of Missouri School of Medicine, Columbia, MO, USA

Teladoc Health Inc., Jefferson City, MO, USA

Alex Rubin Department of Psychology, University of Denver, Denver, CO, USA

Donna A. Ruch Center for Suicide Prevention and Research, Abigail Wexner Research Institute at Nationwide Children's Hospital, Columbus, OH, USA

Arielle H. Sheftall The Center for Suicide Prevention and Research at the Abigail Wexner Research Institute at Nationwide Children's Hospital, Department of Pediatrics at the Ohio State University Medical Center, Columbus, OH, USA

Diana M. Y. Smith Department of Psychology, University of Denver, Denver, CO, USA

Barbara Stanley New York State Psychiatric Institute, New York, NY, USA

Department of Psychiatry, Columbia University Irving Medical Center, New York, NY, USA

Glenn V. Thomas Big Lots Behavioral Health Services, Nationwide Children's Hospital, Columbus, OH, USA

Department of Psychiatry & Behavioral Health, The Ohio State University College of Medicine, Columbus, OH, USA

Sarah Van Norden Spacial Sciences Institute, University of Southern California, Los Angeles, CA, USA

Pankhuree Vandana Nationwide Children's Hospital, Columbus, OH, USA

The Ohio State University, Columbus, OH, USA

Shirley B. Wang Department of Psychology, Harvard University, Cambridge, MA, USA

Holly C. Wilcox Johns Hopkins Bloomberg School of Public Health, Baltimore, MD, USA

Johns Hopkins School of Medicine, Baltimore, MD, USA

Rowan Willis-Powell On Our Own of Maryland, Inc., MD, USA

Jacqueline Wynn Nationwide Children's Hospital, Columbus, OH, USA

The Ohio State University, Columbus, OH, USA

Lucas Zullo Department of Psychiatry and Biobehavioral Sciences, University of California, Los Angeles, CA, USA

Part I
Foundations of Youth Suicide Prevention

Chapter 1
Epidemiology of Suicide and Suicidal Behavior in Youth

Donna A. Ruch and Jeffrey A. Bridge

Suicide is the second leading cause of death among youth aged 10–19 years in the United States (Centers for Disease Control and Prevention [CDC], 2020a). Following a steady decline since 1999, suicide rates in this age group increased 47% between 2010 and 2019 (from 4.2 to 6.6 per 100,000) (CDC, 2020b). The loss of a young life to suicide is a tragic event, leaving a lasting and devastating impact on families, friends, and communities. Although research has advanced many effective strategies to prevent youth suicide, continued efforts are needed to address this pressing public health problem.

Suicidal ideation, defined as thoughts of ending one's life, and suicide attempts, nonfatal self-injurious behavior with stated or inferred intent to die, are also common among youth and some of the strongest predictors of future suicide (O'Carroll et al., 1996). According to the 2019 Youth Risk Behavior Survey (YRBS), completed anonymously by US high school students, 1 in 5 youth indicated they had seriously considered suicide, and 1 out of 11 youth reported they attempted suicide at least once in the prior 12 months (CDC, 2020c). These numbers suggest that healthcare systems and schools should not only seek to identify youth at risk for suicide, but they should also be prepared to support them in a timely and compassionate manner. Numerous risk factors are associated with suicide and suicidal

D. A. Ruch (✉)
Center for Suicide Prevention and Research, Abigail Wexner Research Institute at Nationwide Children's Hospital, Columbus, OH, USA
e-mail: Donna.Ruch@nationwidechildrens.org

J. A. Bridge
Center for Suicide Prevention and Research, Abigail Wexner Research Institute at Nationwide Children's Hospital, Columbus, OH, USA

Departments of Pediatrics, Psychiatry & Behavioral Health, The Ohio State University College of Medicine, Columbus, OH, USA
e-mail: jeff.bridge@nationwidechildrens.org

© The Author(s) 2022
J. P. Ackerman, L. M. Horowitz (eds.), *Youth Suicide Prevention and Intervention*, SpringerBriefs in Psychology,
https://doi.org/10.1007/978-3-031-06127-1_1

behavior including individual (e.g., psychopathology, prior suicidal behavior), family (e.g., familial suicide, family discord, child maltreatment), and social (e.g., school-/peer-related problems) characteristics (Cha et al., 2018). This chapter will focus on recent developments in the epidemiology of youth suicide including trends in demographic subgroups and related risk factors. Knowledge of the complex interplay of factors contributing to youth suicide is highly relevant to the development of effective prevention strategies. Therefore, this chapter seeks to set a foundation of suicide epidemiology for the other chapters in this volume.

Age/Sex

Developmental differences among youth influence the expression and rates of suicidal thoughts and behaviors. Youth suicide rates increase with age, and males are more likely to die by suicide than females (Fig. 1.1). Between 2000 and 2019, youth suicide rates in males were three times higher than females and represented 77% of all suicide deaths in youth aged 10–19 years (CDC, 2020b). However, recent data reveals a narrowing gap between male and female youth suicide rates and age-related sex disparities, with a larger relative increase in suicide rates among younger youth compared to older youth, especially in females (CDC, 2020b). Suicide rates among youth aged 10–14 years increased 100% between 2010 and 2019 (from 1.3 to 2.6 per 100,000), compared to a 40% increase in youth aged 15–19 years (from 7.5 to 10.5 per 100,000) (CDC, 2020b). Suicide rates in females aged 10–14 years showed the sharpest increase, with rates more than doubling during this timeframe (from 0.9 to 2.0 per 100,000; CDC, 2020b). Data further indicate a shift toward a

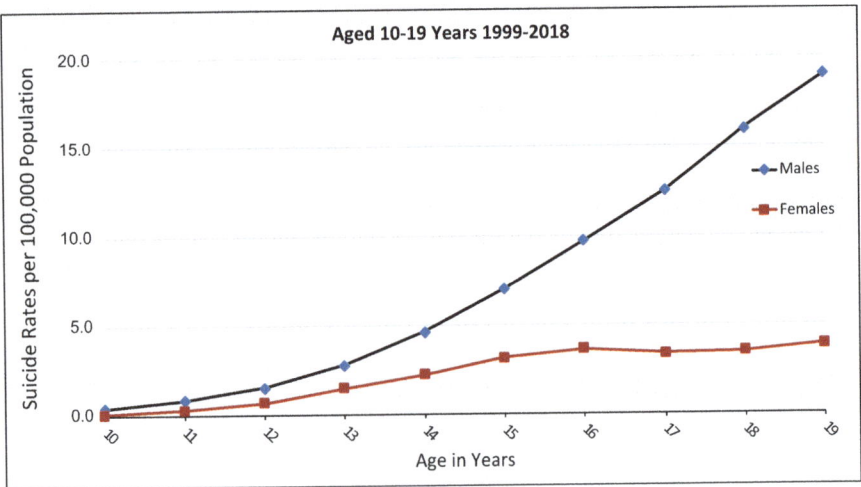

Fig. 1.1 Suicide rates among youth aged 10–19. Suicide rates are displayed by sex (male and female). (Author's own creation)

more highly lethal method of suicide by hanging/suffocation in female youth, which could contribute to the observed increase in female suicide rates (CDC, 2020a). These findings potentially challenge the existing sex-related paradox of youth suicidal behavior, where suicide rates are higher among males than females, yet females have higher rates of suicidal ideation and attempted suicide (Schrijvers et al., 2012).

Race/Ethnicity

Studies also reflect racial and ethnic disparities in rates of suicide and suicidal behavior among youth. American Indian/Alaska Native (AI/AN) youth in the United States have the highest rates of suicide (CDC, 2020b; see also Cwik et al., Chap. 16, this volume). In 2019, the age-adjusted suicide rate among AI/AN youth aged 10–19 years in the United States (23.6 per 100,000) was nearly 3 times the rate for White youth (7.7 per 100,000) and over 4 times higher than rates for Black, Asian/Pacific Islander, and Hispanic youth (CDC, 2020b). Differences by race and ethnicity have also been identified in suicide rates among younger children. An analysis by Bridge et al. (2018) found the suicide rate in children younger than 13 years to be roughly two times higher for Black children compared with White children. An additional study examining suicidal behaviors among US high school students from 1991 to 2017 showed a significant increase in reported suicide attempts by Black youth, while finding no change for White youth, and a significant decrease for all other racial/ethnic groups (Lindsey et al., 2019).

Sexual and Gender Minority Youth

Sexual and gender minority youth are at greater risk for suicide than their peers, even after controlling for other known risk factors (Raifman et al., 2020; Johns et al., 2020; see also Rubin et al., Chap. 13, this volume). Data from the YRBS revealed significantly more sexual minority than heterosexual youth reported suicidal ideation (46.8% vs. 14.5%), a suicide plan (40.2% vs. 12.1%), and at least one suicide attempt (23.4% vs. 6.4%) in the past year (CDC, 2020c). Raifman et al. (2020) evaluated youth sexual orientation and suicide attempts among US high school students and found the proportion of youth reporting any same-sex sexual contact increased by 70%, from 7.7% in 2009 to 13.1% in 2017. Suicide attempt rates decreased in students identifying as sexual minorities during this period, but these students remained more than three times as likely to attempt suicide compared to heterosexual students in 2017 (Raifman et al., 2020). An additional study examined differences in risk and protective factors for suicidal ideation and suicide attempts among sexual minority subgroups in youth aged 12–17 years (Horwitz et al., 2021). Bisexual youth were associated with significantly more suicide risk factors (depression, trauma, victimization) and less protective factors (parent-family connectedness, positive affect), along with elevated rates of both ideation and attempts compared to heterosexual and other sexual minority youth.

Suicide Method

The most common suicide method among US youth aged 10–19 years has historically been by firearms, followed by hanging/suffocation and self-poisoning (CDC, 2020a). This trend has changed in recent years, partially attributable to increases in rates of suicide by hanging/suffocation. Although suicide rates by hanging/suffocation have increased in both males and females, the most notable increase occurred in females aged 10–14 years, with rates more than doubling from 0.66 per 100,000 in 2010 to 1.4 per 100,000 in 2019 (CDC, 2020b; Ruch et al., 2019). Knowledge of method trends can inform targeted community suicide prevention efforts.

Psychopathology

Although many environmental and social factors contribute to suicide risk, research consistently identifies a significant association between youth suicide and mental health, most commonly anxiety, mood, attention, behavior, and behavior disorders (Perou et al., 2013; Ghandour et al., 2019). Comorbidity of mental health issues and substance abuse disorders are also shown to significantly increase the risk for youth suicide and suicidal behavior (Goldston et al., 2009). Notably, depression is strongly linked to youth suicidal thoughts and behaviors (Nock et al., 2013). Results from a national survey show the percentage of youth aged 12–17 years who experienced a past year major depressive episode increased from 9% in 2004 to 15.7% in 2019 (SAMHSA, 2020). In a study comparing suicidal behavior and non-suicidal behavior in youth with mental health conditions, a depression diagnosis was associated with a sixfold greater likelihood of suicidal ideation and attempts, independent of other diagnoses (Nock et al., 2013).

Previous suicidal behavior is one of the most significant predictors of a future suicide attempt (Horwitz et al., 2015; Czyz & King, 2015). In a longitudinal study among youth receiving psychiatric emergency services, a history of suicide attempt was associated with a 4.8-fold increase for future attempts in an 18-month follow-up period (Horwitz et al., 2015). A subsequent study of 13–17-year-olds hospitalized for suicidal behavior found youth with persistent suicidal ideation in the 12 months after discharge were two times as likely to attempt suicide relative to youth whose suicidal ideation declined (Czyz & King, 2015). These findings point to the critical role of transition planning and a continuum of suicide care post-hospitalization for high-risk youth (see Thomas et al., Chap. 15, this volume).

Alcohol/Substance Abuse

Alcohol and substance abuse disorders contribute substantially to the risk for youth suicide (McManama et al., 2014; Liu et al., 2014). In a study of youth aged 12–15 years, alcohol use did not differentiate suicidal youth from non-suicidal youth; however, relative to youth with suicidal ideation, youth who attempted suicide had significantly more frequent alcohol use (McManama et al., 2014). Illicit drug use is also shown to significantly increase the risk for suicide attempts among youth, as well as the transition from ideation to attempt (Liu et al., 2014; Gobbi et al., 2019). In a study examining suicide attempts in intravenous and non-intravenous illicit drug users aged 12–17 years, the odds of suicide attempt were three times as high among youth with a history of using by injection, compared to those who used the same substances through different methods (Liu et al., 2014).

Family Factors

Several family-related factors have been linked to youth suicide. A prospective study examining the familial transmission of suicidal behavior revealed offspring of parents with a history of mood disorders and suicide attempts had a fivefold increased odds of suicide attempt (Brent et al., 2015). An additional study of children aged 9–10 years found family conflict and low parental monitoring were significantly associated with suicidal ideation even after controlling for demographic and psychosocial variables (DeVille et al., 2020).

Studies further indicate parental loss from death, divorce, or abandonment increases the risk for suicide. In a sample of high school-aged youth, Timmons et al. (2011) examined the association between suicide attempts, feelings of belonging, and parental displacement, defined as a separation from parents or substantial disruption in the parent/child relationship. Results showed youth who experienced parental displacement and low feelings of belonging had the highest rates of suicide attempts (Timmons et al., 2011).

A large body of research suggests child maltreatment is a significant risk for youth suicide (Angelakis et al., 2020; Cha et al., 2018; Gomez et al., 2017). A study in youth aged 13–18 years found experiences of childhood abuse were associated with a 5.1 and 5.8 increase in suicidal ideation and attempt, respectively (Gomez et al., 2017), while a meta-analysis examining child maltreatment and youth suicidal behavior found sexual abuse was the most significant predictor of suicidal behavior (Angelakis et al., 2020). Youth with a history of sexual abuse were four times more likely to attempt suicide compared to youth who experienced other forms of abuse or neglect (Angelakis et al., 2020).

Bullying

Bullying victimization and offending have also been identified as important risk factors for youth suicide (Koyanagi et al., 2019; Alavi et al., 2017). Using data from 48 countries, a global study found bullying victimization was associated with a threefold increased odds for a suicide attempt among youth aged 12–15 years (Koyanagi et al., 2019). An additional study assessed bullying and suicidal ideation in patients aged 12–17 years presenting to an emergency department with mental health issues (Alavi et al., 2017). Slightly more than 75% of youth indicated they experienced bullying at some point during their lives. Findings further revealed that victims of bullying were nine times more likely to report suicidal ideation than youth with no history of bullying (Alavi et al., 2017).

Media/Social Media Effects

There is increasing evidence that time youth spend online and using social media can influence suicidal behavior but that these associations are complex. Duration of use and how content is engaged by youth is highly relevant. A systematic review investigating social media/internet use and suicide attempts in youth aged 11–18 years found more frequent social media/internet use was associated with increased odds (1.03–5.10) for suicide attempt (Sedgwick et al., 2019). The same review highlighted cyberbullying and sleep disturbance as potential mediating factors for this association. In an additional review, up to 25% of studies suggested positive aspects of social media/internet use, revealing youth with a history of suicidal behavior used the internet as a form of support and sense of community to seek help and connect with others (Marchant et al., 2017).

Another concern is media contagion effects, referring to the media's direct and indirect influence on youth suicidal behavior. Recent studies indicate that sensational reports on the suicide of a celebrity that disregard reporting guidelines (Niederkrotenthaler et al., 2020) and irresponsible fictional accounts of suicide such as those found in 13 Reasons Why Season 1 (Bridge et al., 2020) may increase the rate of suicides in the population. Dunlop et al. (2011) examined contagion effects associated with online platforms and whether internet sites and social media exposed youth to information that might increase suicidal ideation. Among youth aged 14–21 years, 79% reported being exposed to suicide-related content through family, friends, and traditional media and 59% through online sources (Dunlop et al., 2011).

Conclusions/Implications

This brief review of epidemiology and recent trends in youth suicide highlights the need for future research aimed at identifying mechanisms related to individual, family, and social influences that increase risk of suicidal thoughts and behavior. Suicide prevention strategies that take both sex and developmental level into consideration and incorporate a culturally informed approach are critical. Evidence further supports the need for prevention efforts that address the distinct needs of sexual and gender minority youth and include improvements in lethal means restriction, abuse prevention, and targeted interventions to improve family and peer relations for vulnerable youth.

While epidemiology has played a critical role in suicide surveillance, risk identification, and intervention development to reduce youth suicide, opportunities exist to advance existing research methods to better inform suicide prevention strategies. Innovative data analytical techniques such as machine learning (see Wang et al., Chap. 3, this volume) and other applications of artificial intelligence are shown to more accurately predict suicide risk and identify individuals at the greatest need for intervention (Navarro et al., 2021; Walsh et al., 2018). Genome-wide association studies also offer a novel approach to suicide risk assessment by potentially detecting genetic variations that contribute to suicidal behavior (Kimbrel et al., 2018; Perlis et al., 2010). Given the recent increases in preteen suicide rates, psychological autopsy studies can provide insight into specific risks associated with this age group to support early intervention (Ruch et al., 2019). Lastly, the field of epidemiology may be uniquely positioned to address health inequities. Future efforts involving more diverse population data and comprehensive healthcare information can help target services for potentially high-risk underserved youth.

Funding Details Dr. Bridge receives research grant funding from the National Institute of Mental Health (NIMH), the Patient-Centered Outcomes Research Institute (PCORI), and the Centers for Disease Control and Prevention (CDC); he is also a member of the Scientific Advisory Board of Clarigent Health.

References

Alavi, N., Reshetukha, T., Prost, E., Antoniak, K., Patel, C., Sajid, S., & Groll, D. (2017). Relationship between bullying and suicidal behaviour in youth presenting to the emergency department. *Journal of the Canadian Academy of Child and Adolescent Psychiatry, 26*(2), 70.

Angelakis, I., Austin, J. L., & Gooding, P. (2020). Association of childhood maltreatment with suicide behaviors among young people: A systematic review and meta-analysis. *JAMA Network Open, 3*(8), e2012563. https://doi.org/10.1001/jamanetworkopen.2020.12563

Brent, D. A., Melhem, N. M., Oquendo, M., Burke, A., Birmaher, B., Stanley, B., Biernesser, C., Keilp, J., Kolko, D., Ellis, S., Porta, G., Zelazny, J., Iyengar, S., & Mann, J. J. (2015). Familial pathways to early-onset suicide attempt: A 5.6-year prospective study. *JAMA Psychiatry, 72*(2), 160–168. https://doi.org/10.1001/jamapsychiatry.2014.2141

Bridge, J. A., Horowitz, L. M., Fontanella, C. A., Sheftall, A. H., Greenhouse, J., Kelleher, K. J., & Campo, J. V. (2018). Age-related racial disparity in suicide rates among US youths from 2001 through 2015. *JAMA Pediatrics, 172*(7), 697–699. https://doi.org/10.1001/jamapediatrics.2018.0399

Bridge, J. A., Greenhouse, J. B., Ruch, D., Stevens, J., Ackerman, J., Sheftall, A. H., Horowitz, L. M., Kelleher, K. J., & Campo, J. V. (2020). Association between the release of Netflix's 13 Reasons Why and suicide rates in the United States: An interrupted time series analysis.

Journal of the American Academy of Child and Adolescent Psychiatry, 59(2), 236–243. https://doi.org/10.1016/j.jaac.2019.04.020

Centers for Disease Control and Prevention (CDC). (2020a, February 20). *WISQARS leading causes of death reports, 1981–2019.* https://webappa.cdc.gov/sasweb/ncipc/leadcaus10_us.html

Centers for Disease Control and Prevention (CDC). (2020b, February 20). *WISQARS fatal injury reports, national, regional and state, 1981–2019.* https://webappa.cdc.gov/sasweb/ncipc/mortrate.html

Centers for Disease Control and Prevention (CDC). (2020c, October 27). *Youth risk behavior survey data summary & trends report 2009–2019.* https://www.cdc.gov/healthyyouth/data/yrbs/yrbs_data_summary_and_trends.htm

Cha, C. B., Franz, P. J., Guzmán, M., Glenn, C. R., Kleiman, E. M., & Nock, M. K. (2018). Annual research review: Suicide among youth–epidemiology, (potential) etiology, and treatment. *Journal of Child Psychology and Psychiatry, 59*(4), 460–482. https://doi.org/10.1111/jcpp.12831

Czyz, E. K., & King, C. A. (2015). Longitudinal trajectories of suicidal ideation and subsequent suicide attempts among adolescent inpatients. *Journal of Clinical Child & Adolescent Psychology, 44*(1), 181–193. https://doi.org/10.1080/15374416.2013.836454

DeVille, D. C., Whalen, D., Breslin, F. J., Morris, A. S., Khalsa, S. S., Paulus, M. P., & Barch, D. M. (2020). Prevalence and family-related factors associated with suicidal ideation, suicide attempts, and self-injury in children aged 9 to 10 years. *JAMA Network Open, 3*(2), e1920956. https://doi.org/10.1001/jamanetworkopen.2019.20956

Dunlop, S. M., More, E., & Romer, D. (2011). Where do youth learn about suicides on the Internet, and what influence does this have on suicidal ideation? *Journal of Child Psychology and Psychiatry, 52*(10), 1073–1080. https://doi.org/10.1111/j.1469-7610.2011.02416.x

Ghandour, R. M., Sherman, L. J., Vladutiu, C. J., Ali, M. M., Lynch, S. E., Bitsko, R. H., & Blumberg, S. J. (2019). Prevalence and treatment of depression, anxiety, and conduct problems in US children. *The Journal of Pediatrics, 206*, 256–267. https://doi.org/10.1016/j.jpeds.2018.09.021

Gobbi, G., Atkin, T., Zytynski, T., Wang, S., Askari, S., Boruff, J., Ware, M., Marmorstein, N., Cipriani, A., Dendukuri, N., & Mayo, N. (2019). Association of cannabis use in adolescence and risk of depression, anxiety, and suicidality in young adulthood: A systematic review and meta-analysis. *JAMA Psychiatry, 76*(4), 426–434. https://doi.org/10.1001/jamapsychiatry.2018.4500

Goldston, D. B., Daniel, S. S., Erkanli, A., Reboussin, B. A., Mayfield, A., Frazier, P. H., & Treadway, S. L. (2009). Psychiatric diagnoses as contemporaneous risk factors for suicide attempts among adolescents and young adults: Developmental changes. *Journal of Consulting and Clinical Psychology, 77*(2), 281. https://doi.org/10.1037/a0014732

Gomez, S. H., Tse, J., Wang, Y., Turner, B., Millner, A. J., Nock, M. K., & Dunn, E. C. (2017). Are there sensitive periods when child maltreatment substantially elevates suicide risk? Results from a nationally representative sample of adolescents. *Depression and Anxiety, 34*(8), 734–741. https://doi.org/10.1002/da.22650

Horwitz, A. G., Czyz, E. K., & King, C. A. (2015). Predicting future suicide attempts among adolescent and emerging adult psychiatric emergency patients. *Journal of Clinical Child & Adolescent Psychology, 44*(5), 751–761. https://doi.org/10.1080/15374416.2014.910789

Horwitz, A. G., Grupp-Phelan, J., Brent, D., Barney, B. J., Casper, T. C., Berona, J., Chernick, L. S., Shenoi, R., Cwik, M., King, C. A., & Pediatric Emergency Care Applied Research Network. (2021). Risk and protective factors for suicide among sexual minority youth seeking emergency medical services. *Journal of Affective Disorders, 279*, 274–281. https://doi.org/10.1016/j.jad.2020.10.015

Johns, M. M., Lowry, R., Haderxhanaj, L. T., Rasberry, C. N., Robin, L., Scales, L., Stone, D., & Suarez, N. A. (2020). Trends in violence victimization and suicide risk by sexual identity among high school students – Youth Risk Behavior Survey, United States, 2015–2019. *MMWR Supplements, 69*(1), 19–27. https://doi.org/10.15585/mmwr.su6901a3

Kimbrel, N. A., Garrett, M. E., Dennis, M. F., Research, V. M. A. M. I., Hauser, M. A., Ashley-Koch, A. E., & Beckham, J. C. (2018). A genome-wide association study of suicide attempts and suicidal ideation in US military veterans. *Psychiatry Research, 269*, 64–69. https://doi.org/10.1016/j.psychres.2018.07.017

Koyanagi, A., Oh, H., Carvalho, A. F., Smith, L., Haro, J. M., Vancampfort, D., Stubbs, B., & DeVylder, J. E. (2019). Bullying victimization and suicide attempt among adolescents aged 12-15 years from 48 countries. *Journal of the American Academy of Child and Adolescent Psychiatry, 58*(9), 907–918.e4. https://doi.org/10.1016/j.jaac.2018.10.018

Lindsey, M. A., Sheftall, A. H., Xiao, Y., & Joe, S. (2019). Trends of suicidal behaviors among high school students in the United States: 1991–2017. *Pediatrics, 144*(5). https://doi.org/10.1542/peds.2019-1187

Liu, R. T., Case, B. G., & Spirito, A. (2014). Injection drug use is associated with suicide attempts but not ideation or plans in a sample of adolescents with depressive symptoms. *Journal of Psychiatric Research, 56*, 65–71. https://doi.org/10.1016/j.jpsychires.2014.05.001

Marchant, A., Hawton, K., Stewart, A., Montgomery, P., Singaravelu, V., Lloyd, K., Purdy, N., Daine, K., & John, A. (2017). A systematic review of the relationship between internet use, self-harm and suicidal behaviour in young people: The good, the bad and the unknown. *PloS One, 12*(8), e0181722. https://doi.org/10.1371/journal.pone.0181722

McManama O'Brien, K. H., Becker, S. J., Spirito, A., Simon, V., & Prinstein, M. J. (2014). Differentiating adolescent suicide attempters from ideators: Examining the interaction between depression severity and alcohol use. *Suicide and Life-Threatening Behavior, 44*(1), 23–33.

Navarro, M. C., Ouellet-Morin, I., Geoffroy, M. C., Boivin, M., Tremblay, R. E., Côté, S. M., & Orri, M. (2021). Machine learning assessment of early life factors predicting suicide attempt in adolescence or young adulthood. *JAMA Network Open, 4*(3), e211450. https://doi.org/10.1001/jamanetworkopen.2021.1450

Niederkrotenthaler, T., Braun, M., Pirkis, J., Till, B., Stack, S., Sinyor, M., & Arendt, F. (2020). Association between suicide reporting in the media and suicide: Systematic review and meta-analysis. *British Medical Journal, 368*, Article m575. https://doi.org/10.1136/bmj.m575

Nock, M. K., Green, J. G., Hwang, I., McLaughlin, K. A., Sampson, N. A., Zaslavsky, A. M., & Kessler, R. C. (2013). Prevalence, correlates, and treatment of lifetime suicidal behavior among adolescents: Results from the National Comorbidity Survey Replication Adolescent Supplement. *JAMA Psychiatry, 70*(3), 300–310. https://doi.org/10.1001/2013.jamapsychiatry.55

O'Carroll, P. W., Berman, A. L., Maris, R. W., Moscicki, E. K., Tanney, B. L., & Silverman, M. M. (1996). Beyond the Tower of Babel: A nomenclature for suicidology. *Suicide and Life-Threatening Behavior, 26*(3), 237–252.

Perlis, R. H., Huang, J., Purcell, S., Fava, M., Rush, A. J., Sullivan, P. F., Hamilton, S. P., McMahon, F. J., Schulze, T. G., Potash, J. B., Zandi, P. P., Willour, V. L., Penninx, B. W., Boomsma, D. I., Vogelzangs, N., Middeldorp, C. M., Rietschel, M., Nöthen, M., Cichon, S., … Smoller, J. W. (2010). Genome-wide association study of suicide attempts in mood disorder patients. *The American Journal of Psychiatry, 167*(12), 1499–1507. https://doi.org/10.1176/appi.ajp.2010.10040541

Perou, R., Bitsko, R. H., Blumberg, S. J., Pastor, P., Ghandour, R. M., Gfroerer, J. C., & Huang, L. N. (2013). Mental health surveillance among children—United States, 2005–2011. *MMWR Supplement, 62*(2), 1–35.

Raifman, J., Charlton, B. M., Arrington-Sanders, R., Chan, P. A., Rusley, J., Mayer, K. H., Stein, M. D., Austin, S. B., & McConnell, M. (2020). Sexual orientation and suicide attempt disparities among US adolescents: 2009–2017. *Pediatrics, 145*(3), e20191658. https://doi.org/10.1542/peds.2019-1658

Ruch, D. A., Sheftall, A. H., Schlagbaum, P., Rausch, J., Campo, J. V., & Bridge, J. A. (2019). Trends in suicide among youth aged 10 to 19 years in the United States, 1975 to 2016. *JAMA Network Open, 2*(5), e193886. https://doi.org/10.1001/jamanetworkopen.2019.3886

Schrijvers, D. L., Bollen, J., & Sabbe, B. G. (2012). The gender paradox in suicidal behavior and its impact on the suicidal process. *Journal of Affective Disorders, 138*(1–2), 19–26. https://doi.org/10.1016/j.jad.2011.03.050

Sedgwick, R., Epstein, S., Dutta, R., & Ougrin, D. (2019). Social media, Internet use and suicide attempts in adolescents. *Current Opinion in Psychiatry, 32*(6), 534. https://doi.org/10.1097/YCO.0000000000000547

Substance Abuse and Mental Health Services Administration (SAMHSA). (2020). *Key substance use and mental health indicators in the United States: Results from the 2019 National Survey on Drug Use and Health.* https://www.samhsa.gov/data/

Timmons, K. A., Selby, E. A., Lewinsohn, P. M., & Joiner, T. E. (2011). Parental displacement and adolescent suicidality: Exploring the role of failed belonging. *Journal of Clinical Child & Adolescent Psychology, 40*(6), 807–817. https://doi.org/10.1080/15374416.2011.614584

Walsh, C. G., Ribeiro, J. D., & Franklin, J. C. (2018). Predicting suicide attempts in adolescents with longitudinal clinical data and machine learning. *Journal of Child Psychology and Psychiatry, 59*(12), 1261–1270. https://doi.org/10.1111/jcpp.12916

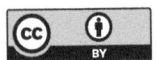

Chapter 2
Neurobiology of Suicide in Children and Adolescents: Implications for Assessment and Treatment

Elizabeth D. Ballard and Maryland Pao

Emergency department visits for youth suicidal thoughts and behaviors are on the rise (Kalb et al., 2019), with the full impact of the recent COVID-19 pandemic on suicide rates still unknown. Given all that is at stake, children and adolescents with suicidal thoughts and behaviors need effective treatments. To maximize their effectiveness, clinicians will benefit from a range of treatments that are rapid, safe, and tailored to the specific clinical and biological needs of each patient. Unfortunately, regardless of age, there are few rapid pharmacologic or non-pharmacologic treatments that have demonstrated immediate or lasting impact on suicidal thoughts and behavior. Options are even more limited for medication treatments for children and adolescents with suicidal thoughts, in part due to understandable concerns around enrolling minors into clinical trials with potentially negative and long-term effects on adolescent physiology and brain development. This cautious approach places clinicians in an untenable situation; they are asked to emergently treat youth with suicidal thoughts and behavior but do not have the requisite clinical tools and evidence-based standards from research. Consequently, clinicians cannot provide many suicidal youth with needed treatments without evidence-based guidance from potentially high-risk research and clinical trials. What follows is an overview of specific neurobiological and pharmacologic research focused on suicide risk and treatment. When possible, we highlight the particular needs of adolescents as distinct from adults in critical areas for future research.

E. D. Ballard (✉)
Section on the Neurobiology and Treatment of Mood Disorders, National Institute of Mental Health, Bethesda, MD, USA
e-mail: elizabeth.ballard@nih.gov

M. Pao
Office of the Clinical Director, National Institute of Mental Health, National Institutes of Health, Bethesda, MD, USA
e-mail: paom@mail.nih.gov

Neurobiological Research of Adolescents at Risk of Suicide

First, any discussion of the neurobiology of suicide in adolescents should consider the role of brain development. The human brain does not fully mature until around age 24 years (Gogtay et al., 2004). Between childhood and adulthood, the adolescent brain undergoes many changes that place adolescents at unique risk for impulsive emotional behavior. For example, the prefrontal cortex (PFC), which is involved in planning, impulse control, and executive functioning, is one of the last brain areas to fully mature and appears to develop at different rates in males and females (Hammerslag & Gulley, 2016). In contrast, limbic regions associated with emotional reactivity, such as the nucleus accumbens and amygdala, are fully matured in adolescence (Casey et al., 2008). Thus, the adolescent brain is "wired" to have strong emotional reactions, particularly to interpersonal interactions, at a time when their ability to plan and control impulses is less developed. This tendency toward reactive behaviors puts adolescents, particularly males, at risk for impulsive suicidal behavior. Research around functional magnetic resonance imaging (fMRI) and adolescent suicide attempters has mostly focused on reactions to emotional stimuli, for example, brain reactivity to perceived angry faces or social exclusion (Harms et al., 2019). Overall, neuroimaging studies suggest that adolescents with a history of suicide attempt show altered neural activity in areas related to emotional processing. One analysis of adolescent suicide attempters, as compared to non-attempters with bipolar disorder, showed reduced functional connectivity between the amygdala (part of limbic system) and PFC associated with suicide attempt lethality and suicide ideation severity (Johnston et al., 2017). Thus, adolescents at highest suicide risk may have altered connectivity between the emotional (limbic) and self-control regions (PFC) of the brain. These changes in brain connectivity represent potential targets for future intervention whether through learning strategies for emotional coping in psychotherapy to strengthen these brain pathways or by impacting the neural connectivity underlying decision-making through pharmacologic or neuromodulation strategies (e.g., transcranial magnetic stimulation (TMS)).

Second, there are genetic influences on suicidal behavior that place certain adolescents at higher risk of suicide. Family studies have indicated that children of parents with a suicide attempt history are at increased likelihood of suicide attempt, possibly due to influence of impulsive aggression, inheritance of mood disorders, or environmental exposures to suicidal behavior (Brent et al., 2015; Kendler et al., 2020). While there is unlikely to be a specific "gene" associated with suicide risk, analyses that take into account the influence of many genes, termed "polygenic risk scores," are currently in use to evaluate the multifactorial impact of genetic risk on suicidal behavior. In one example, polygenic risk scores for bipolar disorder predicted risk for suicide attempt in a sample of adolescents and young adults but only in the context of a traumatic stress history (Wilcox et al., 2017). Clearly, both genetic and environmental factors interact in the development of adolescent suicidal behavior within families. These factors suggest possible opportunities for targeted intervention. For example, future programs could treat offspring of parents who attempt suicide to determine whether such intervention impacts later suicidal thoughts and behaviors, particularly for individuals with both parental suicidal behavior and traumatic event experiences.

The next generation of interventions based on current neurobiological research suggests that it may be important to intervene with certain patient groups *before* they make their first suicide attempt, namely, individuals with impulsivity or familial suicidal behavior. Additionally, it will be critical to understand the behavioral manifestations of these neurobiological markers. For example, adolescents with altered connectivity between emotional and self-control regions of the brain could be evaluated using technologies such as ecological momentary assessment (EMA), which typically involves the repeated assessment of current experiences on smartphone devices (Shiffman et al., 2008), in order to obtain a "real-time" observation of emotional reactivity and impulsivity. Similarly, individuals with parental suicidal behavior could be evaluated using measures of implicit suicide risk, which assess biases toward death and suicide-related stimuli (Nock et al., 2010). By incorporating these exciting new technologies with neurobiological measures, researchers can target their treatments to where it is most needed in order to prevent later suicidal behavior (see also Wang et al., Chap. 3, this volume).

Barriers and Opportunities for Pharmacologic Treatment

Clinical trials for suicide risk are critical but difficult to conduct due to ethical and clinical concerns of enrolling and monitoring individuals at risk for suicide. These concerns are further compounded in trials involving adolescents due to concerns about minor assent/parent consent, adherence to treatment regimens, the possible negative impact of interventions on brain development and long-term consequences, as well as the aforementioned tendency of adolescents to engage in impulsive behavior. As such, adequately powered studies designed to evaluate pharmacologic treatment outcomes for suicidal adolescents are uncommon. The following section discusses two areas relevant to expanding opportunities for effective pharmacologic treatment: (1) understanding the impact of the selective serotonin reuptake inhibitor (SSRI) "black box" warning for suicide risk and (2) strategies to expand emerging research.

In the early 2000s, the US Food and Drug Administration (FDA) received reports from pharmaceutical companies that SSRIs, commonly prescribed for depression, were associated with increased risk of suicide attempt in adolescents. These reports led to further FDA investigation and a 2004 black box warning for the use of SSRIs in children and adolescents, due to concerns for suicide risk in youth up to 24 years of age with clear drug efficacy in older adults (for a full account of the FDA evaluation, please see Hammad et al., 2006). This black box warning has been associated with significant controversy; reanalysis of the randomized clinical trial (RCT) data by different groups has reported inconsistent results and questionable coding of suicidal thoughts and behaviors (Posner et al., 2007). What is known is that antidepressant prescription rates for children and adolescents sharply fell after this warning (Lu et al., 2014). This drop in prescriptions has been linked to increased adolescent suicide rates suggesting that depressed and suicidal adolescents were no longer receiving needed treatments, although there is also contentious debate about this relationship (Gibbons et al., 2007). Delineating the underlying relationship between SSRIs and suicide is well beyond the scope of this review but does highlight the following principles: (1) a positive relationship between SSRIs and suicide risk is not found for adults, emphasizing the need to evaluate the efficacy and safety of pharmacologic treatments in adolescent samples; and (2) prescribing any psychiatric medication to a child or adolescent requires careful monitoring and extensive documentation, particularly in the first few weeks of treatment. One major concern is that the SSRI black box warning has deterred further pharmacologic investigations into suicide-focused treatments especially for youth. Sadly, research in adult depression clinical trials has suggested that individuals with suicidal thoughts and behaviors are also now more likely be excluded from research (Zimmerman et al., 2015), even as suicide rates continue to increase. We propose that suicide-focused clinical trials in adolescents are needed now more than ever and that concerns around the need for enhanced observation, assessment, and media scrutiny do not outweigh the benefits of preventing death by suicide.

In the absence of such evidence-based treatments, clinicians may consider other off-label treatments. Clozapine, the only FDA-approved medication for the treatment of suicide attempt, is primarily prescribed for the treatment of schizophrenia, has several major side effects, and is rarely used in children and adolescents. Lithium has been associated with reduced suicide attempt rates and aggression in a sample of children and adolescents with bipolar disorder, (Hafeman et al., 2020) but is not FDA approved for suicidal behavior in any age group. Newer treatments, ketamine and transcranial magnetic stimulation (TMS), are currently being evaluated for adults; if effective, these will require careful additional evaluation in adolescent populations. Ketamine has a history of being used medically as a dissociative anesthetic but also as a drug of abuse. Subanesthetic intravenous administrations of ketamine are associated with transient reductions in suicidal thoughts within minutes to hours. Initial open-label trials of ketamine have been conducted in adolescents (Cullen et al., 2018), but research is proceeding with understandable caution due to concerns of substance abuse and potential effects on the developing adolescent brain. Even with a sufficient evidence base, a provider might weigh the benefits of transient relief of intractable suicidal thoughts and depression in an at-risk youth with concerns that the individual might then pursue further ketamine administrations to the detriment of other effective pharmacologic and non-pharmacologic therapies. Similarly, TMS involves the noninvasive direct stimulation of the brain using magnetic pulses. While there is an established literature on TMS for depression, which has recently expanded to include initial open-label trials of TMS in adolescents with depression and suicidal thoughts, concerns remain about permanent neural alterations (Croarkin et al., 2018). Therefore, while promising treatments may be on the horizon, clinicians treating at-risk youth have limited pharmacologic resources at their disposal and often must weigh the concerns of treating imminent suicide risk with off-label use of psychiatric medications without a clear evidence base.

Comprehensive evidence-based guidelines for the treatment of children and adolescents with suicidal thoughts and behaviors are essential. Carefully designed and monitored clinical trials of treatments such as lithium, ketamine, and TMS in adolescents could inform future prescribing practices to understand which individuals are most likely to benefit from which treatments as well as potential side effects. Since it is likely that most youth with suicidal thoughts and behaviors are prescribed medications off-label, standardized patient registries and protocols may be needed for a complete understanding of the potential effects (and unintended side effects) of these treatments. In short, more data on the effects of pharmacologic treatments for adolescents at risk for suicide is necessary for clinicians to aid their clinical decision-making.

Conclusions and Policy Recommendations

Adolescence represents a critical period in development during which the brain is most reactive to emotional stimuli but vulnerable due to underdeveloped planning and impulse control. Furthermore, genetic predisposition and environmental stressors can put an adolescent at additional risk for suicide. Due to key brain changes that occur over the course of early development, it cannot be assumed that treatments for suicide that are efficacious for adults will show similar effects in adolescents. In addition, because of safety concerns, clinical treatment trials in adolescents have been limited. As such, it is likely that suicidal adolescents are undertreated, resulting in a clear call-to-action to develop research studies and clinical trials focused on neurobiological risk factors and treatment targets in adolescents. First, neurobiological research points to areas of intervention *before* a child or adolescent makes a first suicide attempt, namely, individuals with impulsivity and/or familial suicide risk. Second, for individuals already experiencing suicidal thoughts and behavior, clinical trials are critically needed to understand which treatments provide the most benefit, potentially incorporating new modes of data collection that monitor real-time active and implicit suicide risk. Policy recommendations include providing guidance to ethical review boards on how to evaluate research and clinical trials with suicidal youth as well as disseminating resources to support psychiatrists and primary care practitioners on the effective treatment of youth at risk for suicide including best practice care pathways and treatment algorithms. Without such research and resources, adolescents with suicidal thoughts and behaviors will continue to be undertreated, putting them at further risk of distress, suicidal behavior, and death.

Funding Details This research was supported in part by the Intramural Research Program of the NIMH (Annual Report Numbers ZIAMH002922 and ZIAMH002927).

References

Brent, D. A., Melhem, N. M., Oquendo, M., Burke, A., Birmaher, B., Stanley, B., Biernesser, C., Keilp, J., Kolko, D., Ellis, S., Porta, G., Zelazny, J., Iyengar, S., & Mann, J. J. (2015). Familial pathways to early-onset suicide attempt: A 5.6-year prospective study. *JAMA Psychiatry, 72*(2), 160–168. https://doi.org/10.1001/jamapsychiatry.2014.2141

Casey, B. J., Jones, R. M., & Hare, T. A. (2008). The adolescent brain. *Annals of the New York Academy of Science, 1124*, 111–126. https://doi.org/10.1196/annals.1440.010

Croarkin, P. E., Nakonezny, P. A., Deng, Z. D., Romanowicz, M., Voort, J. L. V., Camsari, D. D., Schak, K. M., Port, J. D., & Lewis, C. P. (2018). High-frequency repetitive TMS for suicidal ideation in adolescents with depression. *Journal of Affective Disorders, 239*, 282–290. https://doi.org/10.1016/j.jad.2018.06.048

Cullen, K. R., Amatya, P., Roback, M. G., Albott, C. S., Westlund Schreiner, M., Ren, Y., Eberly, L. E., Carstedt, P., Samikoglu, A., Gunlicks-Stoessel, M., Reigstad, K., Horek, N., Tye, S., Lim, K. O., & Klimes-Dougan, B. (2018). Intravenous ketamine for adolescents with treatment-resistant depression: An open-label study. *Journal of Child Adolescent Psychopharmacology, 28*(7), 437–444. https://doi.org/10.1089/cap.2018.0030

Gibbons, R. D., Brown, C. H., Hur, K., Marcus, S. M., Bhaumik, D. K., Erkens, J. A., Herings, R. M., & Mann, J. J. (2007). Early evidence on the effects of regulators' suicidality warnings on SSRI prescriptions and suicide in children and adolescents. *American Journal of Psychiatry, 164*(9), 1356–1363. https://doi.org/10.1176/appi.ajp.2007.07030454

Gogtay, N., Giedd, J. N., Lusk, L., Hayashi, K. M., Greenstein, D., Vaituzis, A. C., Nugent, T. F., 3rd, Herman, D. H., Clasen, L. S., Toga, A. W., Rapoport, J. L., & Thompson, P. M. (2004). Dynamic mapping of human cortical development during childhood through early adulthood. *Proceedings of the National Academy of Sciences of the United States of America, 101*(21), 8174–8179. https://doi.org/10.1073/pnas.0402680101

Hafeman, D. M., Rooks, B., Merranko, J., Liao, F., Gill, M. K., Goldstein, T. R., Diler, R., Ryan, N., Goldstein, B. I., Axelson, D. A., Strober, M., Keller, M., Hunt, J., Hower, H., Weinstock, L. M., Yen, S., & Birmaher, B. (2020). Lithium versus other mood-stabilizing medications in a longitudinal study of youth diagnosed with bipolar disorder. *Journal of the American Academy of Child and Adolescent Psychiatry, 59*(10), 1146–1155. https://doi.org/10.1016/j.jaac.2019.06.013

Hammad, T. A., Laughren, T., & Racoosin, J. (2006). Suicidality in pediatric patients treated with antidepressant drugs. *Archives of General Psychiatry, 63*(3), 332–339. https://doi.org/10.1001/archpsyc.63.3.332

Hammerslag, L. R., & Gulley, J. M. (2016). Sex differences in behavior and neural development and their role in adolescent vulnerability to substance use. *Behavioural Brain Research, 298*(Pt A), 15–26. https://doi.org/10.1016/j.bbr.2015.04.008

Harms, M. B., Casement, M. D., Teoh, J. Y., Ruiz, S., Scott, H., Wedan, R., & Quevedo, K. (2019). Adolescent suicide attempts and ideation are linked to brain function during peer interactions. *Psychiatry Research Neuroimaging, 289*, 1–9. https://doi.org/10.1016/j.pscychresns.2019.05.001

Johnston, J. A. Y., Wang, F., Liu, J., Blond, B. N., Wallace, A., Liu, J., Spencer, L., Cox Lippard, E. T., Purves, K. L., Landeros-Weisenberger, A., Hermes, E., Pittman, B., Zhang, S., King, R., Martin, A., Oquendo, M. A., & Blumberg, H. P. (2017). Multimodal neuroimaging of fron-tolimbic structure and function associated with suicide attempts in adolescents and young adults with bipolar disorder. *American Journal of Psychiatry, 174*(7), 667–675. https://doi.org/10.1176/appi.ajp.2016.15050652

Kalb, L. G., Stapp, E. K., Ballard, E. D., Holingue, C., Keefer, A., & Riley, A. (2019). Trends in psychiatric emergency department visits among youth and young adults in the US. *Pediatrics, 143*(4). https://doi.org/10.1542/peds.2018-2192

Kendler, K. S., Ohlsson, H., Sundquist, J., Sundquist, K., & Edwards, A. C. (2020). The sources of parent-child transmission of risk for suicide attempt and deaths by suicide in Swedish national samples. *American Journal of Psychiatry, 177*(10), 928–935. https://doi.org/10.1176/appi.ajp.2020.20010017

Lu, C. Y., Zhang, F., Lakoma, M. D., Madden, J. M., Rusinak, D., Penfold, R. B., Simon, G., Ahmedani, B. K., Clarke, G., Hunkeler, E. M., Waitzfelder, B., Owen-Smith, A., Raebel, M. A., Rossom, R., Coleman, K. J., Copeland, L. A., & Soumerai, S. B. (2014). Changes in antidepressant use by young people and suicidal behavior after FDA warnings and media coverage: Quasi-experimental study. *British Medical Journal, 348*, g3596. https://doi.org/10.1136/bmj.g3596

Nock, M. K., Park, J. M., Finn, C. T., Deliberto, T. L., Dour, H. J., & Banaji, M. R. (2010). Measuring the suicidal mind: Implicit cognition predicts suicidal behavior. *Psychological Science, 21*(4), 511–517. https://doi.org/10.1177/0956797610364762

Posner, K., Oquendo, M. A., Gould, M., Stanley, B., & Davies, M. (2007). Columbia classification algorithm of suicide assessment (C-CASA): Classification of suicidal events in the FDA's pediatric suicidal risk analysis of antidepressants. *American Journal of Psychiatry, 164*(7), 1035–1043. https://doi.org/10.1176/ajp.2007.164.7.1035

Shiffman, S., Stone, A. A., & Hufford, M. R. (2008). Ecological momentary assessment. *Annual Review of Clinical Psychology, 4*, 1–32. https://doi.org/10.1146/annurev.clinpsy.3.022806.091415

Wilcox, H. C., Fullerton, J. M., Glowinski, A. L., Benke, K., Kamali, M., Hulvershorn, L. A., Stapp, E. K., Edenberg, H. J., Roberts, G. M. P., Ghaziuddin, N., Fisher, C., Brucksch, C., Frankland, A., Toma, C., Shaw, A. D., Kastelic, E., Miller, L., McInnis, M. G., Mitchell, P. B., & Nurnberger, J. I., Jr. (2017). Traumatic stress interacts with bipolar disorder genetic risk to increase risk for suicide attempts. *Journal of the American Academy of Child and Adolescent Psychiatry, 56*(12), 1073–1080. https://doi.org/10.1016/j.jaac.2017.09.428

Zimmerman, M., Clark, H. L., Multach, M. D., Walsh, E., Rosenstein, L. K., & Gazarian, D. (2015). Have treatment studies of depression become even less generalizable? A review of the inclusion and exclusion criteria used in placebo-controlled antidepressant efficacy trials published during the past 20 years. *Mayo Clinic Proceedings, 90*(9), 1180–1186. https://doi.org/10.1016/j.mayocp.2015.06.016

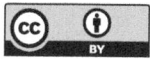

Chapter 3
Machine Learning for Suicide Prediction and Prevention: Advances, Challenges, and Future Directions

Shirley B. Wang, Walter Dempsey, and Matthew K. Nock

In the 50 years from 1965 to 2015, researchers published over 350 papers examining variables that might enhance the prediction of youth suicidal thoughts and behaviors (STBs). Unfortunately, a meta-analysis of this work found predictive accuracy has *not* increased over time, but rather, it has remained just slightly above chance for all outcomes (Franklin et al., 2017). One possible explanation is that the vast majority of studies have focused on single risk factors from the same few domains (e.g., mental health) combined in simple ways (e.g., multiple linear regression) across extended timeframes (e.g., >10 years). To address these limitations, researchers recently have turned to novel machine learning methods, which can model high-dimensional datasets with potentially complex nonlinear relationships among risk factors and outcomes. These studies have so far demonstrated superior performance of machine learning compared to traditional statistical methods (Linthicum et al., 2019). For instance, machine learning models have provided high accuracy in predicting suicide attempts in large, nationally representative surveys (García de la Garza et al., 2021), US Army soldiers (Kessler et al., 2017), and patients hospitalized for suicidal thoughts and behaviors (Wang et al., 2021). However, several outstanding questions remain regarding how to best build and implement machine learning models to guide clinical decision-making. In this chapter, we discuss key challenges at each step of the research process to provide recommendations for researchers, clinicians, and policy makers interested in machine learning for youth suicide prevention. Of note, we focus on broad, higher-level concepts throughout this chapter, rather than technical aspects of

S. B. Wang (✉) · M. K. Nock
Department of Psychology, Harvard University, Cambridge, MA, USA
e-mail: shirleywang@g.harvard.edu; nock@wjh.harvard.edu

W. Dempsey
Department of Biostatistics, University of Michigan, Ann Arbor, MI, USA
e-mail: wdem@umich.edu

© The Author(s) 2022
J. P. Ackerman, L. M. Horowitz (eds.), *Youth Suicide Prevention
and Intervention*, SpringerBriefs in Psychology,
https://doi.org/10.1007/978-3-031-06127-1_3

implementation and analysis, and direct interested readers to recent tutorials and textbooks for greater technical detail (Dwyer et al., 2018; Kuhn & Johnson, 2013).

Important Questions and Challenges

Data Collection

How researchers collect data influences the effectiveness of STB prediction. Choices made during data collection can significantly impact a model's accuracy. For instance, models using predictors that are *causes* of the outcome may be more deployable in other sites than models with predictors that are *effects* of the outcome (Piccininni et al., 2020), though model adjustments also remain important if site populations are very different from one another. In addition to predictor selection, researchers should carefully consider the timeframes of interest. Most existing youth STB prediction models have considered long follow-up periods (an average of 7.9 years for adolescents; Franklin et al., 2017), which do not reflect the time-frame of greatest clinical interest (i.e., risk of a patient attempting suicide in the next few days, weeks, or months), especially during periods of rapid emotional and cog-nitive development. Recent research harnessing advances in smartphone and wear-able biosensor technology has enabled shorter-term risk prediction during these critical time periods (e.g., following psychiatric hospitalization) (Wang et al., 2021) demonstrating that despite the time- and effort-intensive nature of real-time moni-toring studies, they can provide important data for STB prediction in high-risk time periods.

Model Building

Numerous machine learning algorithms have been applied in STB prediction, including regularized regression (e.g., elastic net), random forests, neural networks, and naive Bayes classifiers. A full review of these models is beyond the scope of this chapter, and we encourage readers to consult excellent reviews (Dwyer et al., 2018) and textbooks (James et al., 2013) for greater technical detail. It is worth noting that each approach has benefits and drawbacks, with complex nonlinear methods (e.g., random forests, neural networks) typically requiring more data to perform well and yielding higher prediction accuracy at the cost of lower interpretability, and vice versa for simpler linear methods (e.g., regularized regression). When choosing an algorithm, researchers should consider their ultimate goals, which could be (1) to maximize accuracy, (2) to interpret the logic of how each variable contributes to the prediction of outcomes, or (3) to identify potential targets for prevention and inter-vention efforts.

Once an algorithm has been selected, an important question is whether to consider missing data as a predictor in the model. Such an informative missingness approach has the potential to pick up on key contributors to suicide risk. For instance, in a sample of nearly 4,000 US Army soldiers, nonresponse to a question about suicidal thinking emerged as a particularly strong predictor of future suicide attempts (Nock et al., 2018). However, researchers should proceed with caution when using missingness as a predictor in machine learning models, as changes to study design would lead to changes in missing data patterns, and some evidence suggests it may also introduce bias into models that generalize poorly to new data (van Smeden et al., 2020). Following these decisions, researchers should split data into training and test datasets to reduce likelihood of overfitting and evaluate accuracy with multiple metrics for a complete understanding of model performance.

Model Implementation and Translation

As our ability to refine predictive models improves, they can be implemented in settings where youth with elevated suicide risk are most likely to present, such as healthcare settings. How models are best implemented is discussed here. Broadly speaking, there are three options. The first involves building a model and applying this exact model to new sites. This often is used for other health outcomes, such as eye diseases, cardiac abnormalities, and cancer (Ngiam & Khor, 2019). Benefits of this approach include faster implementation and model dissemination, while drawbacks include less tailoring to site characteristics that could influence predictive accuracy (e.g., population health status, prescribing patterns, billing code assignments). Another approach involves using the same modeling *approach* but training a new model at each new site. Across five US healthcare systems, a recent study using this approach found remarkably consistent accuracy for predicting suicide attempts (Barak-Corren et al., 2020). The third option offers a compromise: rather than build entirely new models or implement identical models across sites, researchers could use existing models to update models for new populations. This could involve shrinkage of a new model toward existing models or using information from previous models as priors at new sites.

A related concern in implementing machine learning models involves temporal drift. For example, it is unknown if a model built in 2020 would show similar accuracy in the same population in 2030. This challenge is perhaps best exemplified by the current worldwide COVID-19 pandemic. Many models built prior to COVID-19 may fail to adequately capture the importance and magnitude of current strong predictors of STBs, such as feelings of isolation (Fortgang et al., 2021). Thus, even after models are implemented clinically, they should be continually updated based on newly available data.

Using Models to Guide Clinical Decision-Making

Healthcare providers must also consider how to integrate information from machine learning models into their decision-making. A critical concern when working with high-risk patients is forecasting risk of suicide to make decisions about clinical care and need for hospitalization. The goal of building and implementing STB prediction models is not to replace clinical judgment, but rather to guide, support, and augment clinical decision-making. For instance, when faced with a decision about whether to hospitalize or discharge a patient who may be at risk for suicide, clinicians could consult predictions from a machine learning model, just as they may consult other members of the clinical care team.

However, two concerns that undermine use of models currently are the high rate of false positives *and* false negatives in STB prediction models to date. The problem of false positives has been noted as early as the 1980s (Pokorny, 1983) and continues to present challenges with integrating machine learning into clinical decision-making today. As psychiatric hospitalization is often the first-line intervention for individuals at imminent suicide risk, high false positive rates could risk unnecessary hospitalization for thousands of patients erroneously predicted to be at acute suicide risk annually. When hospitalization occurs in the absence of clinical need, this can have serious iatrogenic effects via increased distress, stigma, trauma (e.g., witnessing threatening/violent behavior from patients or staff), coercion, and loss of autonomy, particularly for involuntary hospitalizations (Ward-Ciesielski & Rizvi, 2020). Many hospitals are already overburdened, and false positives may compromise a hospital's ability to meet the needs of true positive cases. Failing to detect acute suicide risk when it exists (e.g., false negatives) is also highly concerning as they represent missed opportunities for timely and potentially lifesaving intervention. In light of these potentials for harm, machine learning models should be used to augment, not replace, clinical decision-making.

Ethics of Machine Learning for Youth Suicide Prediction

Accurate prediction of youth suicide is only useful insofar as there are effective STB prevention strategies. Unfortunately, we currently lack strong and universally effective interventions (Fox et al., 2020), and the common intervention of hospitalization has serious potential harms, including high suicide risk post-discharge. Crucially, we do not know if psychiatric hospitalization helps more people than it harms nor the precise effectiveness of hospitalization in preventing suicide (Large & Kapur, 2018). Thus, alongside research optimizing machine learning algorithms for STB prediction, there is a critical need to develop and disseminate effective and scalable STB interventions, particularly for youth (see Thomas et al., Chap. 15, this volume; Zullo et al., Chap. 8, this volume).

Regardless of these limitations, researchers and clinicians must know how to respond if a child or adolescent is predicted to be at high suicide risk. A recent Delphi study by Nock et al. (2021) including scientists, clinicians, ethicists, legal experts, and individuals with lived experience provided a consensus statement that individuals identified in a research context to be at high risk for suicide should (1) be contacted as soon as possible (including contact with parents), (2) receive an individualized safety plan, (3) receive additional risk assessment, and (4) receive personalized outreach rather than automated contact. Importantly, many experts discouraged calling 911 as a standard response, as police contact can result in elevated rates of physical force, trauma, and death, particularly for racial or ethnic minorities (Nock et al., 2021). We also note that simply contacting people predicted to be at high suicide risk is itself an intervention, the effects of which are unknown and worth investigating. Although this Delphi study was conducted in the context of real-time monitoring research studies, many principles may apply to ethical concerns of machine learning risk predictions. We encourage researchers, clinicians, and policy makers to continually update best-practice guidelines over time as more data and considerations become available.

Future Directions

In this chapter, we have outlined critical unanswered questions at every stage of the process from building to implementing machine learning models for youth suicide prevention. Clearly, there is much work to be done, and we believe that expertise is needed from multiple domains and perspectives, including psychology, psychiatry, and clinical practitioners, in addition to computer scientists, statisticians, ethicists, and those with lived experience. Collaborative science is essential for making meaningful progress especially in the challenging arena of predicting suicide risk.

In addition to data-driven machine learning methods, we also note the importance of strong theory in advancing STB prediction and prevention. Although there are many influential suicide theories, these have all been instantiated *verbally*, which renders them underspecified due to the inherent imprecision of language. Formalizing theories using mathematical and computational modeling can advance the prediction and prevention of suicide by identifying factors *causally* associated with STBs and potential targets for intervention (which can also be simulated to understand if, how, and why a treatment may be effective for reducing suicide risk).

Both theory- and data-driven computational work are crucial for youth STB prevention. Machine learning has revolutionized many fields of medicine over the past decade. To make similar progress, we need a better understanding of the causes of STBs, the effect of model predictions on clinical decision-making, external validation of models, best-practice ethical guidelines, and effective and scalable interventions. In addition, greater funding for suicide research is crucial for driving innovation and exploring the challenges described above. Whereas increased federal funding has led to declines in other leading causes of death (e.g., tuberculosis) over the past century, funding for suicide research has lagged far behind, and the suicide rate today is nearly identical to what it was 100 years ago (Fortgang & Nock, 2021). Increased funding and policy to support continued research in prediction of youth suicide can provide critical information to inform the development and implementation of machine learning models to meaningfully reduce suicide in youth.

Funding Details Shirley Wang is supported by the National Science Foundation Graduate Research Fellowship under Grant No. DGE-1745303 and the National Institute of Mental Health under Grant F31MH125495. Walter Dempsey is supported by the National Institute of Drug Abuse under Grants R01DA039901 and P50DA054039.

References

Barak-Corren, Y., Castro, V. M., Nock, M. K., Mandl, K. D., Madsen, E. M., Seiger, A., Adams, W. G., Applegate, R. J., Bernstam, E. V., Klann, J. G., McCarthy, E. P., Murphy, S. N., Natter, M., Ostasiewski, B., Patibandla, N., Rosenthal, G. E., Silva, G. S., Wei, K., Weber, G. M., … Smoller, J. W. (2020). Validation of an electronic health record–based suicide risk prediction modeling approach across multiple health care systems. *JAMA Network Open, 3*(3), e201262. https://doi.org/10.1001/jamanetworkopen.2020.1262

Dwyer, D. B., Falkai, P., & Koutsouleris, N. (2018). Machine learning approaches for clinical psychology and psychiatry. *Annual Review of Clinical Psychology, 14*(1), 91–118. https://doi.org/10.1146/annurev-clinpsy-032816-045037

Fortgang, R. G., & Nock, M. K. (2021). Ringing the alarm on suicide prevention: A call to action. *Psychiatry, 84*(2), 192–195. https://doi.org/10.1080/00332747.2021.1907871

Fortgang, R. G., Wang, S. B., Millner, A. J., Reid-Russell, A., Beukenhorst, A. L., Kleiman, E. M., Bentley, K. H., Zuromski, K. L., Al-Suwaidi, M., Bird, S. A., Buonopane, R., DeMarco, D., Haim, A., Joyce, V. W., Kastman, E. K., Kilbury, E., Lee, H.-I. S., Mair, P., Nash, C. C., … Nock, M. K. (2021). Increase in suicidal thinking during COVID-19. *Clinical Psychological Science, 9*, 482–488. https://doi.org/10.1177/2167702621993857

Fox, K. R., Huang, X., Guzmán, E. M., Funsch, K. M., Cha, C. B., Ribeiro, J. D., & Franklin, J. C. (2020). Interventions for suicide and self-injury: A meta-analysis of randomized controlled trials across nearly 50 years of research. *Psychological Bulletin*. https://doi.org/10.1037/bul0000305

Franklin, J. C., Ribeiro, J. D., Fox, K. R., Bentley, K. H., Kleiman, E. M., Huang, X., Musacchio, K. M., Jaroszewski, A. C., Chang, B. P., & Nock, M. K. (2017). Risk factors for suicidal thoughts and behaviors: A meta-analysis of 50 years of research. *Psychological Bulletin, 143*(2), 187–232. https://doi.org/10.1037/bul0000084

García de la Garza, Á., Blanco, C., Olfson, M., & Wall, M. M. (2021). Identification of suicide attempt risk factors in a national US survey using machine learning. *JAMA Psychiatry, 78*(4), 398–406. https://doi.org/10.1001/jamapsychiatry.2020.4165

James, G., Witten, D., Hastie, T., & Tibshirani, R. (2013). *An introduction to statistical learning* (Vol. 103). Springer. https://doi.org/10.1007/978-1-4614-7138-7

Kessler, R. C., Stein, M. B., Petukhova, M. V., Bliese, P., Bossarte, R. M., Bromet, E. J., Fullerton, C. S., Gilman, S. E., Ivany, C., Lewandowski-Romps, L., Bell, A. M., Naifeh, J. A., Nock, M. K., Reis, B. Y., Rosellini, A. J., Sampson, N. A., Zaslavsky, A. M., & Ursano, R. J. (2017). Predicting suicides after outpatient mental health visits in the army study to assess risk and resilience in servicemembers (Army STARRS). *Molecular Psychiatry, 22*(4), 544–551. https://doi.org/10.1038/mp.2016.110

Kuhn, M., & Johnson, K. (2013). *Applied predictive modeling*. Springer-Verlag. https://doi.org/10.1007/978-1-4614-6849-3

Large, M. M., & Kapur, N. (2018). Psychiatric hospitalisation and the risk of suicide. *The British Journal of Psychiatry, 212*(5), 269–273. https://doi.org/10.1192/bjp.2018.22

Linthicum, K. P., Schafer, K. M., & Ribeiro, J. D. (2019). Machine learning in suicide science: Applications and ethics. *Behavioral Sciences & the Law, 37*(3), 214–222. https://doi.org/10.1002/bsl.2392

Ngiam, K. Y., & Khor, I. W. (2019). Big data and machine learning algorithms for health-care delivery. *The Lancet Oncology, 20*(5), e262–e273. https://doi.org/10.1016/S1470-2045(19)30149-4

Nock, M. K., Millner, A. J., Joiner, T. E., Gutierrez, P. M., Han, G., Hwang, I., King, A., Naifeh, J. A., Sampson, N. A., Zaslavsky, A. M., Stein, M. B., Ursano, R. J., & Kessler, R. C. (2018). Risk factors for the transition from suicide ideation to suicide attempt: Results from the army study to assess risk and resilience in servicemembers (Army STARRS). *Journal of Abnormal Psychology, 127*(2), 139–149. https://doi.org/10.1037/abn0000317

Nock, M. K., Kleiman, E. M., Abraham, M., Bentley, K. H., Brent, D. A., Buonopane, R. J., Castro-Ramirez, F., Cha, C. B., Dempsey, W., Draper, J., Glenn, C. R., Harkavy-Friedman, J., Hollander, M. R., Huffman, J. C., Lee, H. I. S., Millner, A. J., Mou, D., Onnela, J.-P., Picard, R. W., ... Pearson, J. L. (2021). Consensus statement on ethical & safety practices for conducting digital monitoring studies with people at risk of suicide and related behaviors. *Psychiatric Research and Clinical Practice, 3*(2), 57–66. https://doi.org/10.1176/appi.prcp.20200029

Piccininni, M., Konigorski, S., Rohmann, J. L., & Kurth, T. (2020). Directed acyclic graphs and causal thinking in clinical risk prediction modeling. *BMC Medical Research Methodology, 20*(1), 179. https://doi.org/10.1186/s12874-020-01058-z

Pokorny, A. D. (1983). Prediction of suicide in psychiatric patients: Report of a prospective study. *Archives of General Psychiatry, 40*(3), 249. https://doi.org/10.1001/archpsyc.1983.01790030019002

van Smeden, M., Groenwold, R. H. H., & Moons, K. G. M. (2020). A cautionary note on the use of the missing indicator method for handling missing data in prediction research. *Journal of Clinical Epidemiology, 125*, 188–190. https://doi.org/10.1016/j.jclinepi.2020.06.007

Wang, S. B., Coppersmith, D. D. L., Kleiman, E. M., Bentley, K. H., Millner, A. J., Fortgang, R., Mair, P., Dempsey, W., Huffman, J. C., & Nock, M. K. (2021). A pilot study using frequent inpatient assessments of suicidal thinking to predict short-term postdischarge suicidal behavior. *JAMA Network Open, 4*(3), e210591. https://doi.org/10.1001/jamanetworkopen.2021.0591

Ward-Ciesielski, E. F., & Rizvi, S. L. (2020). The potential iatrogenic effects of psychiatric hospitalization for suicidal behavior: A critical review and recommendations for research. *Clinical Psychology: Science and Practice*, e12332. https://doi.org/10.1111/cpsp.12332

Part II
Suicide Prevention and Postvention in School Settings

Chapter 4
Effective Suicide Prevention and Intervention in Schools

Lynsay Ayer, Kerri Nickerson, Julie Goldstein Grumet, and Sharon Hoover

Suicide is a complex public health issue that requires the implementation of multiple interventions to address the constellation of risk and protective factors that may exist in students' lives. The school setting provides numerous opportunities for contribution to a comprehensive multi-tiered approach to suicide prevention, especially for youth who reside in communities with limited mental health resources. The implementation of such school-based suicide prevention efforts advances a culture of care that encourages help-seeking and connectedness among youth. While schools are often limited by budget and staffing constraints, collaborations with state and local partners, including health and behavioral health systems, can help to mitigate these barriers. This chapter outlines key elements of a comprehensive strategy to address suicide prevention and mental health promotion in schools.

Dr. Lynsay Ayer contributed to this work during the scope of her employment at the RAND Corporation. Therefore, this is considered "work made for hire" and the authorized RAND representative has signed the agreement.

L. Ayer (✉)
RAND Corporation, Arlington, VA, USA
e-mail: layer@rand.org

K. Nickerson
American Institutes for Research, Arlington, VA, USA
e-mail: knickerson@edc.org

J. G. Grumet
Education Development Center, Waltham, MA, USA
e-mail: JGoldstein@edc.org

S. Hoover
National Center for School Mental Health, University of Maryland, College Park, MD, USA
e-mail: shoover@som.umaryland.edu

Evidence-based interventions and recommendations for practice and future research are highlighted.

A Comprehensive Strategy for School-Based Suicide Prevention

Growing evidence shows that comprehensive suicide prevention programs involving a variety of interventions that address multiple risk and protective factors for suicide may reduce suicide rates (Garraza et al., 2019; Knox et al., 2010; Stone et al., 2017). Three primary approaches, when used together, have the potential to reduce suicidal behaviors: (1) *prevention*, implementation of upstream interventions that support mental health promotion, foster the development of healthy coping strategies and connectedness among the entire school community, and encourage help-seeking when mental health concerns arise; (2) *early identification*, to identify students who may be at risk for suicide and establish clear protocols for how to respond when a student is identified as being at risk; and (3) *response*, to adopt strategies to connect students at risk for suicide with evidence-based, culturally appropriate care and respond to the needs of the school community when a student dies by suicide. In this chapter we provide an overview of the evidence in these areas but refer readers to recent reviews and meta-analyses (Brann et al., 2020; Singer et al., 2019) for more detailed discussions of the evidence regarding specific school-based suicide prevention programs and the strengths and limitations of each.

Prevention

Population-based interventions that address healthy coping strategies and life skill development, including those targeting elementary school classrooms, are particularly effective at reducing suicide (Wilcox et al., 2008; Wyman, 2014). For example, the Good Behavior Game (Barrish et al., 1969) is a program designed to promote positive social skills and effective coping behavior in classrooms and has been shown to reduce suicidal ideation later in life (Wilcox et al., 2008). The Youth Aware of Mental Health (YAM; Wasserman et al., 2015) program is an evidence-based universal program that educates high school students about mental health as well as risk and protective factors for suicide and provides them with skills to manage distress and suicidal behavior. In a cluster-randomized controlled trial, YAM prevented suicide attempts at a 12-month follow-up assessment (Wasserman et al., 2015). For a comprehensive list of suicide prevention programs available to schools, the Suicide Prevention Resource Center has a searchable database of school-based suicide prevention programs (SPRC, 2021). Additionally, the Substance Abuse and Mental Health Services Administration has published a toolkit for comprehensive suicide prevention in high schools (SAMHSA, 2012).

Schools should consider the various cultures of their students and families when identifying effective and meaningful interventions to support the development of healthy coping strategies and life skills. One example of a culturally grounded intervention is American Indian Life Skills, which has shown promise in reducing feelings of hopelessness, a risk factor for suicide (LaFromboise & Howard-Pitney, 1995). More work is needed to increase the application of suicide prevention in culturally responsive ways.

Schools can also play an important role in encouraging healthy, open, and transparent discussions among students and school staff about mental health and the importance of talking to a trusted adult or peer when needed (Goldston et al., 2010). Many schools have done this through communication campaigns (e.g., public service announcements, posters, social media campaigns). Although the literature base for the efficacy of suicide prevention communication materials lacks rigor, a systematic review revealed some evidence that media campaigns can positively influence student help-seeking behaviors, improve suicide awareness among students, and potentially even reduce number of suicides (Pirkis et al., 2019).

Early Identification

A key component of any comprehensive suicide prevention strategy is to proactively identify students who are at increased risk for suicide. Importantly, asking students about suicidal thoughts does not increase distress or cause harm such as increased suicidal ideation or behavior (Gould et al., 2005; Polihronis et al., 2020). Two common methods include screening for suicide risk and implementing training programs to help school community members identify and appropriately respond to and refer a student who is at risk for suicide.

Both universal and targeted screening can be conducted in schools (see Mournet et al., Chap. 7, this volume). Universal screening involves administering a screening tool to an entire grade or school, regardless of individuals' level of risk. By contrast, in a targeted screening approach, the screening tool is only administered to students who have known or emerging risk factors (e.g., history of suicidal behavior, talking about suicide or displaying warning signs, recent significant loss). The 11-item Columbia-Suicide Severity Rating Scale (CSSR-S), Ask Suicide-Screening Questions (ASQ), and Patient Health Questionnaire-9 modified for Adolescents (PHQ-A) are examples of tools that are commonly used in schools and medical settings to detect suicide risk among adolescents (Horowitz et al., 2009). Several studies have concluded that school-based screening for suicide risk identifies at-risk students who would not have been otherwise identified by school professionals (Gould et al., 2009; Scott et al., 2009). It is important to note that the validity of suicide risk screening tools for children under 10 years has not been established and tools developed for older youth may not be appropriate for younger children (Ayer et al., 2020). However, school staff can be trained to recognize warnings signs for younger children (e.g., talking about wanting to die, engaging in self-injurious behaviors, displaying severe depressive symptoms, etc.) and refer them for further mental health assessment. Whenever there is a concern about suicide risk (based on the child's words or behavior, no matter the age of the child), the child should be referred for immediate follow-up with a trained professional.

Training programs that provide information about suicide warning signs and how to respond if these signs are identified are often called "gatekeeper trainings." Gatekeeper training programs typically train non-clinicians, in this case the students, parents, and/or school staff such as teachers, coaches, and office staff, to recognize and respond to students at risk for suicide. Gatekeeper programs with empirical support include Signs of Suicide and Sources of Strength, which have reported increases in help-seeking behaviors, improved perceptions of adult support options, and some evidence that they reduce student suicide attempts (see Ackerman et al., Chap. 5, this volume; Schilling et al., 2016; Wyman et al., 2010). Furthermore, promoting a school culture where school community members are able to openly discuss mental health and suicide risk may help to foster student belonging, connectedness, and community-level emotional support which are key protective factors for adolescent suicide (Whitlock et al., 2014).

Overall, research is still limited on the impact of gatekeeper training on student suicide risk (Yonemoto et al., 2019). Specifically, while initial evidence suggests that it can improve trainees' knowledge and confidence in identifying and responding to those at risk for suicide (Garraza et al., 2019), there is little evidence that this translates to behavior change in adults or students (Robinson-Link et al., 2019; Yonemoto et al., 2019) in a sustained manner.

Response to Student Suicide Risk

Once a student is identified as at risk for suicide, steps must be taken to conduct a more in-depth assessment of suicide risk, engage caregivers, and connect the student with evidence-based, culturally responsive care. Challenges can arise when mental health resources are not readily available to support individuals identified through early identification and assessment. Brief suicide safety assessment tools that help triage next steps for students that screen positive include the ASQ BSSA (National Institute of Mental Health, 2020) and the C-SSRS (Posner et al., 2011). It is critical that schools assess the availability of mental health resources – either within the school or in the community – prior to setting up a screening program. Additionally, schools should have a protocol for following up with students who screen positive and/or are referred for additional services to ensure that barriers are navigated, the referral appointment occurs, and the care transition is supported. Finally, schools should ensure that all staff are knowledgeable of the existing crisis protocol with defined roles for who responds to a student after disclosure of suicidal ideation or behavior, who notifies parents, and what follow-up will occur.

Safety planning is a key aspect of a response to any person at risk for suicide, and there are evidence-based protocols for conducting safety planning with adolescents at high risk for suicide (Czyz et al., 2019; see Monahan & Stanley, Chap. 9, this volume). One example of an evidence-based safety planning intervention is the Stanley-Brown Safety Plan (Stanley & Brown, 2011). A strengths-based collaborative safety plan should be developed for any student who expresses thoughts of suicide with the goal of empowering the student to delay action in suicidal thoughts by considering accessible alternatives to self-harm. The safety plan should be developed on the same day the student screens positive for suicide, updated frequently, and should be shared with all providers as part of continuity of care.

A response to youth suicide risk may include inpatient or outpatient mental health treatment, including interventions offered directly in the school building. There is compelling evidence that children and adolescents are significantly more likely to initiate and complete evidence-based behavioral health interventions offered in schools compared to other community mental health settings (Jaycox et al., 2010). Some schools may be able to integrate programs that have been shown to reduce youth suicide risk in other settings (e.g., medical settings or homes). For example, a variety of family-based programs, such as the Family Bereavement Program and Family Check-Up, that were originally focused on reducing risk factors for suicide (e.g., substance use, mental health symptoms) can also reduce or prevent youth suicidal ideation while simultaneously impacting their original treatment targets (Reider & Sims, 2016). Programs like these, which have "crossover" or "spillover" effects on suicide risk, can be an efficient way for schools to address multiple behavioral health concerns. Schools with greater capacity for mental health services may be able to integrate programs like these, while others may find it most efficient to develop strong partnerships and referral pathways with community mental health providers to whom students can be referred.

Schools should also be prepared to respond in the event a suicide death occurs within their school community, otherwise known as postvention (see Diefendorf et al., Chap. 6, this volume). When a student dies of suicide, the school needs to respond in a timely, effective way that inhibits the spread of misinformation, providing information about normal responses to grief and loss and where to access resources. For example, the American Foundation for Suicide Prevention (AFSP) and SPRC created the "After a Suicide" toolkit to guide high schools in responding to a suicide loss (AFSP, 2018).

Opportunities for Action

Addressing suicide in schools can feel daunting, especially in the face of resource constraints and competing priorities. This chapter highlighted key components of a comprehensive strategy for school-based suicide prevention and identified practices with scientific support, as well as many areas in need of further, more rigorous research. To maximize schools' potential for success, we offer the following recommendations:

1. Early, universal prevention is a worthy investment. Although more research is needed, evidence suggests that the implementation of such programs (e.g., in elementary school) has the potential to reduce risk for not only suicide, but other adverse outcomes like drug and alcohol misuse and emotional and behavioral problems. Therefore, these early prevention programs may have a higher likelihood of impact and prove cost-effective for schools in the long run.

2. Consider cultural factors in any school-based suicide prevention research, policy, or practice. While we know that some youth populations are at higher risk for suicide (e.g., AI/AN and LGBTQ youth), many suicide prevention programs are developed, tested, and implemented without sufficient consideration of how programs could be enhanced or adapted to be more inclusive, culturally responsive, and effective for these more vulnerable populations (see Chu & Khoury, Chap. 11, this volume). Self-reported suicide attempts have been rising among Black youth even as attempts by other groups have declined suggesting the need to focus additional attention and resources on Black youth as well (see Sheftall & Boyd, Chap. 12, this volume). With so much work yet to be done on school-based suicide prevention, these considerations must not be an afterthought, but should be "baked into" any suicide prevention effort.

3. Schools should evaluate the impact of their suicide prevention programs, whether new or existing. As we and others (e.g., Katz et al., 2013) have highlighted, there is an urgent need for more data on the outcomes of suicide prevention practices in schools. Information about how programs impact student suicidal ideation and behavior is particularly valuable. Attention to fidelity and implementation of evidence-based models is also warranted (see Ackerman et al., Chap. 5, this volume). Evaluation efforts including randomized controlled trials may require additional funding and collaboration with outside partners such as academic researchers, local medical or mental health providers, and strong relationships with school districts.

4. Researchers should examine whether other school-based mental health initiatives and social emotional learning (SEL) programs have "spillover" effects on student suicide risk. With major, national movements supporting trauma-informed schools and SEL more generally, there may be opportunities to add measures of suicidal risk to examine whether such programs also impact suicidal ideation and behavior. For instance, youth exposed to trauma like child abuse and neglect are at risk for suicide; therefore, school-based programs intended to mitigate traumatic stress in this group may also prevent suicide. Promising universal SEL programs such as DBT STEPS-A (Mazza & Dexter-Mazza, 2019) offer students the opportunity to learn the types of individual and interpersonal coping skills that are effective in mitigating a suicidal crisis.

5. Researchers should work with practitioners and school mental health partners to develop suicide risk screening and assessment approaches for students as early as elementary school and test their validity and reliability, as well as feasibility and acceptability in school settings. Evidence-based guidance for identifying and managing suicide risk in very young students is lacking, despite concerning

increases in suicide among minoritized youth (Ayer et al., 2020; Lindsey et al., 2019).

6. Studies on how to effectively implement safety planning in schools are needed. Safety planning is an important piece of any suicide prevention effort, but most of the research on this approach comes from clinical settings (e.g., Czyz et al., 2019). Implementation studies on how to adapt safety planning for the school context and for youth of differing developmental abilities are needed to inform the use of this approach.

Conclusions

Schools are uniquely positioned to prevent youth suicide. There is a consensus in the field that a comprehensive approach to suicide prevention is the best way to prevent suicide, identify students at risk, and respond appropriately. Researchers and policymakers can contribute to advancing the science, practice, and policies that are still emerging. Specifically, policy interventions may include mandatory annual or biannual gatekeeper trainings for school staff, mandatory prevention programming or screening initiatives at certain grade levels, and training requirements for school-based mental health providers. Though additional research is needed to strengthen the evidence for these practices, schools can and should adopt thoughtful approaches to suicide risk identification and care that build connectedness, train staff to respond, and ultimately link youth to quality care.

Acknowledgments The authors would like to thank Shawn Orenstein, MPH, for her comments on previous versions of this chapter.

References

American Foundation for Suicide Prevention. (2018). *After a suicide: A toolkit for schools, second edition.* https://www.sprc.org/resources-programs/after-suicide-toolkit-schools. Accessed 16 Sept 2021.

Ayer, L., Colpe, L., Pearson, J., Rooney, M., & Murphy, E. (2020). Advancing research in child suicide: A call to action. *Journal of the American Academy of Child and Adolescent Psychiatry, 59*(9), 1028–1035. https://doi.org/10.1016/j.jaac.2020.02.010

Barrish, H. H., Saunders, M., & Wolf, M. M. (1969). Good behavior game: Effects of individual contingencies for group consequences on disruptive behavior in a classroom. *Journal of Applied Behavior Analysis, 2*(2), 119–124. https://doi.org/10.1901/jaba.1969.2-119

Brann, K. L., Baker, D., Smith-Millman, M. K., Watt, S. J., & DiOrio, C. (2020). A meta-analysis of suicide prevention programs for school-aged youth. *Children and Youth Services Review,* 105826. https://doi.org/10.1016/j.childyouth.2020.105826

Czyz, E. K., King, C. A., & Biermann, B. J. (2019). Motivational interviewing-enhanced safety planning for adolescents at high suicide risk: A pilot randomized controlled trial. *Journal of

Clinical Child and Adolescent Psychology, 48(2), 250–262. https://doi.org/10.1080/1537441
6.2018.1496442

Godoy Garraza, L., Kuiper, N., Goldston, D., McKeon, R., & Walrath, C. (2019). Long-term impact of the Garrett Lee Smith Youth Suicide Prevention Program on youth suicide mortality, 2006-2015. *Journal of Child Psychology and Psychiatry, and Allied Disciplines, 60*(10), 1142–1147. https://doi.org/10.1111/jcpp.13058

Goldston, D. B., Walrath, C. M., McKeon, R., Puddy, R. W., Lubell, K. M., Potter, L. B., & Rodi, M. S. (2010). The Garrett Lee Smith memorial suicide prevention program. *Suicide & Life-Threatening Behavior, 40*(3), 245–256. https://doi.org/10.1521/suli.2010.40.3.245

Gould, M. S., Marrocco, F. A., Kleinman, M., Thomas, J. G., Mostkoff, K., Cote, J., & Davies, M. (2005). Evaluating iatrogenic risk of youth suicide screening programs: A randomized controlled trial. *JAMA, 293*(13), 1635–1643. https://doi.org/10.1001/jama.293.13.1635

Gould, M. S., Marrocco, F. A., Hoagwood, K., Kleinman, M., Amakawa, L., & Altschuler, E. (2009). Service use by at-risk youths after school-based suicide screening. *Journal of the American Academy of Child and Adolescent Psychiatry, 48*(12), 1193–1201. https://doi.org/10.1097/CHI.0b013e3181bef6d5

Horowitz, L. M., Ballard, E. D., & Pao, M. (2009). Suicide screening in schools, primary care and emergency departments. *Current Opinion in Pediatrics, 21*(5), 620–627. https://doi.org/10.1097/MOP.0b013e3283307a89

Jaycox, L. H., Cohen, J. A., Mannarino, A. P., Walker, D. W., Langley, A. K., Gegenheimer, K. L., Scott, M., & Schonlau, M. (2010). Children's mental health care following Hurricane Katrina: A field trial of trauma-focused psychotherapies. *Journal of Traumatic Stress, 23*(2), 223–231. https://doi.org/10.1002/jts.20518

Katz, C., Bolton, S. L., Katz, L. Y., Isaak, C., Tilston-Jones, T., Sareen, J., & Swampy Cree Suicide Prevention Team. (2013). A systematic review of school-based suicide prevention programs. *Depression and anxiety, 30*(10), 1030–1045. https://doi.org/10.1002/da.22114

Knox, K. L., Pflanz, S., Talcott, G. W., Campise, R. L., Lavigne, J. E., Bajorska, A., … Caine, E. D. (2010). The US Air Force suicide prevention program: Implications for public health policy. *American Journal of Public Health, 100*(12), 2457–2463. https://doi.org/10.2105/AJPH.2009.159871

LaFromboise, T., & Howard-Pitney, B. (1995). The Zuni life skills development curriculum: Description and evaluation of a suicide prevention program. *Journal of Counseling Psychology, 42*(4), 479.

Lindsey, M. A., Sheftall, A. H., Xiao, Y., & Joe, S. (2019). Trends of suicidal behaviors among high school students in the United States: 1991–2017. *Pediatrics, 144*(5), e20191187. https://doi.org/10.1542/peds.2019-1187

Mazza, J. J., & Dexter-Mazza, E. T. (2019). DBT skills in schools: Implementation of the DBT steps – A social emotional curriculum. In M. A. Swales (Ed.), *The Oxford handbook of dialectical behaviour therapy* (pp. 719–733). Oxford University Press.

National Institute of Mental Health. (2020). *Ask Suicide-Screening Questions (ASQ) toolkit.* www.nimh.nih.gov/ASQ. Accessed 26 Jan 2022.

Pirkis, J., Rossetto, A., Nicholas, A., Ftanou, M., Robinson, J., & Reavley, N. (2019). Suicide prevention media campaigns: A systematic literature review. *Health Communication, 34*(4), 402–414. https://doi.org/10.1080/10410236.2017.1405484

Polihronis, C., Cloutier, P., Kaur, J., Skinner, R., & Cappelli, M. (2020). What's the harm in asking? A systematic review and meta-analysis on the risks of asking about suicide-related behaviors and self-harm with quality appraisal. *Archives of Suicide Research*, 1–23. https://doi.org/10.1080/13811118.2020.1793857

Posner, K., Brown, G. K., Stanley, B., Brent, D. A., Yershova, K. V., Oquendo, M. A., Currier, G. W., Melvin, G. A., Greenhill, L., Shen, S., & Mann, J. J. (2011). The Columbia-suicide severity rating scale: Initial validity and internal consistency findings from three multisite studies with adolescents and adults. *The American Journal of Psychiatry, 168*(12), 1266–1277. https://doi.org/10.1176/appi.ajp.2011.10111704

Reider, E., & Sims, B. (2016). Family-based preventative interventions: Can the onset of suicide ideation and behavior be prevented? *Suicide & Life-Threatening Behavior, 46*, S3–S7. https://doi.org/10.1111/sltb.12252

Robinson-Link, N., Hoover, S., Bernstein, L., Lever, N., Maton, K., & Wilcox, H. (2019). Is gatekeeper training enough for suicide prevention? *School Mental Health, 12*, 239–249.

Schilling, E. A., Aseltine, R. H., Jr., & James, A. (2016). The SOS Suicide Prevention Program: Further evidence of efficacy and effectiveness. *Prevention Science, 17*(2), 157–166. https://doi.org/10.1007/s11121-015-0594-3

Scott, M. A., Wilcox, H. C., Schonfeld, I. S., Davies, M., Hicks, R. C., Turner, J. B., & Shaffer, D. (2009). School-based screening to identify at-risk students not already known to school professionals: The Columbia suicide screen. *American Journal of Public Health, 99*(2), 334–339. https://doi.org/10.2105/AJPH.2007.127928

Singer, J. B., Erbacher, T. A., & Rosen, P. (2019). School-based suicide prevention: A framework for evidence-based practice. *School Mental Health, 11*(1), 54–71. https://doi.org/10.1007/s12310-018-9245-8

Stanley, B., & Brown, G. K. (2011). Safety planning intervention: A brief intervention to mitigate suicide risk. *Cognitive and Behavioral Practice, 19*, 256–264. https://doi.org/10.1016/j.cbpra.2011.01.001

Stone, D., Holland, K., Bartholow, B., Crosby, A., Davis, S., & Wilkins, N. (2017). *Preventing suicide: A technical package of policy, programs, and practices.* Centers for Disease Control and Prevention. https://www.cdc.gov/violenceprevention/pdf/suicideTechnicalPackage.pdf?s_cid=cs_293

Substance Abuse and Mental Health Services Administration (SAMHSA). (2012). *Preventing suicide: A toolkit for high schools.* https://store.samhsa.gov/product/Preventing-Suicide-A-Toolkit-for-High-Schools/SMA12-4669

Suicide Prevention Resource Center (SPRC). (2021). *Resources and programs.* https://www.sprc.org/resources-programs. Accessed 16 Sept 2021.

Wasserman, D., Hoven, C. W., Wasserman, C., Wall, M., Eisenberg, R., Hadlaczky, G., Kelleher, I., Sarchiapone, M., Apter, A., Balazs, J., Bobes, J., Brunner, R., Corcoran, P., Cosman, D., Guillemin, F., Haring, C., Iosue, M., Kaess, M., Kahn, J. P., … Carli, V. (2015). School-based suicide prevention programmes: The SEYLE cluster-randomised, controlled trial. *Lancet (London, England), 385*(9977), 1536–1544. https://doi.org/10.1016/S0140-6736(14)61213-7

Whitlock, J., Wyman, P. A., & Moore, S. R. (2014). Connectedness and suicide prevention in adolescents: Pathways and implications. *Suicide & Life-Threatening Behavior, 44*(3), 246–272. https://doi.org/10.1111/sltb.12071

Wilcox, H. C., Kellam, S. G., Brown, C. H., Poduska, J. M., Ialongo, N. S., Wang, W., & Anthony, J. C. (2008). The impact of two universal randomized first- and second-grade classroom interventions on young adult suicide ideation and attempts. *Drug and Alcohol Dependence, 95*, S60–S73. https://doi.org/10.1016/j.drugalcdep.2008.01.005

Wyman, P. A. (2014). Developmental approach to prevent adolescent suicides: Research pathways to effective upstream preventive interventions. *American Journal of Preventive Medicine, 47*(3), S251–S256. https://doi.org/10.1016/j.amepre.2014.05.039

Wyman, P. A., Brown, C. H., LoMurray, M., Schmeelk-Cone, K., Petrova, M., Yu, Q., Walsh, E., Tu, X., & Wang, W. (2010). An outcome evaluation of the Sources of Strength suicide prevention program delivered by adolescent peer leaders in high schools. *American Journal of Public Health, 100*(9), 1653–1661. https://doi.org/10.2105/AJPH.2009.190025

Yonemoto, N., Kawashima, Y., Endo, K., & Yamada, M. (2019). Gatekeeper training for suicidal behaviors: A systematic review. *Journal of Affective Disorders, 246*, 506–514. https://doi.org/10.1016/j.jad.2018.12.052

Chapter 5
Implementation and Dissemination Strategies for School-Based Suicide Prevention Programs

John P. Ackerman, Oula Khoury, and Samanta Boddapati

Suicide is the second leading cause of death among school-aged youth aged 10–19, and the sharpest increase in number of suicides occurs between early adolescence and young adulthood. Moreover, the majority of those who have ever considered or attempted suicide first did so during their youth (Nock et al., 2013). Ayer and colleagues (Chap. 4, this volume) emphasize that schools provide a context for meaningful suicide prevention activity. Effective school-based suicide prevention programs modify school culture, enhance connectedness, and improve student help-seeking attitudes while reducing mental health stigma. Suicide prevention programs in schools can reduce self-reported suicidal behavior among students and improve school staff confidence and competence in identifying and supporting students at risk for suicide (Aseltine et al., 2007; Wasserman et al., 2015). However, if programming is time-limited or fails to attend to the local needs of the community, benefits do not extend beyond a year or two (Garraza et al., 2019). Faced with limited resources, schools often use a piecemeal approach to prevention, reducing the effectiveness and level of sustainability necessary to maintain reductions in student

J. P. Ackerman (✉) · S. Boddapati
Big Lots Behavioral Health Services, Nationwide Children's Hospital, Columbus, OH, USA

Department Psychiatry & Behavioral Health, The Ohio State University College of Medicine, Columbus, OH, USA
e-mail: john.ackerman@nationwidechildrens.org;
Samanta.Boddapati@nationwidechildrens.org

O. Khoury
Big Lots Behavioral Health Services, Nationwide Children's Hospital, Columbus, OH, USA

Department of Pediatrics, The Ohio State University College of Medicine, Columbus, OH, USA
e-mail: oula.khoury@nationawidechildrens.org

© The Author(s) 2022
J. P. Ackerman, L. M. Horowitz (eds.), *Youth Suicide Prevention and Intervention*, SpringerBriefs in Psychology,
https://doi.org/10.1007/978-3-031-06127-1_5

suicidal behaviors. Schools and communities need to know not only what programs work but how to implement those programs for them to take root and fit into an existing array of supports.

This chapter highlights the role of implementation science and quality improvement strategies to improve school engagement, staff buy-in, and program sustainability. We discuss the role of hospital-school-community partnerships in enhancing the delivery of upstream suicide prevention efforts using the PAX Good Behavior Game (elementary) and the SOS Signs of Suicide Prevention Program (secondary) as examples. We highlight gaps in research regarding the effectiveness of suicide prevention programs as well as ideal dissemination strategies. Recommendations are provided to support how schools and communities can maximize implementation and sustainability.

Implementation Science Framework

It is important to frame our discussion with a few basic assumptions drawn from the implementation science literature. First, suicide prevention efforts should have clearly operationalized outcomes, and programs need to be tested rigorously to gauge effectiveness of implementation in the real world. Suicide prevention knowledge and attitude improvements are important in assessing a program's relative value, but a change in student and staff behaviors should also be prioritized by evaluation (e.g., increased help-seeking behaviors and linkage rates or reduced suicide attempts, hospital admissions, and suicide deaths). Second, prevention program outcomes tend to be positively linked with implementation fidelity (Durlak & Dupre, 2008). Implementation fidelity, or the degree to which a program is implemented as planned and originally evaluated, requires that programs have well-articulated core elements that can be replicated by schools. However, it is also necessary to balance program fidelity with flexibility as perfect implementation fidelity is unrealistic in school settings. Taking an overly rigid or prescriptive approach may inadvertently reduce program adoption and ownership by schools. Furthermore, states differ in requirements and support for mental health programming, which may present both opportunities and barriers. Prevention programming should match local needs to maximize school engagement and effectiveness. Lastly, sustainability should be part of planning from the very beginning. Shared decision-making with partners from the school community is critical to buy-in. Empowering local leadership is needed to drive a lasting culture shift around mental health in schools.

Challenges and Opportunities in Schools

Currently, there are few universal youth suicide prevention programs that have been rigorously evaluated using randomized control trials (RCTs) with strong statistical controls. Furthermore, many outcome evaluations fail to use valid and reliable outcome measures, engage in external peer review processes, or replicate findings (see Miller et al., 2009). Often programs promote certain "active ingredients" thought to be necessary to improve individual or school-level outcomes, but data are unsuited to confirm or refute potential mechanisms of change. Despite these limitations, there are processes known to enhance implementation of suicide prevention efforts which include the following: (1) assessing school needs and readiness for program implementation, (2) developing a strong infrastructure (e.g., hospital-school-community partnerships), (3) building capacity in the school while providing technical assistance, and (4) maintaining fidelity while focusing on program sustainability.

School Readiness for Suicide Prevention

Although schools represent a setting well situated to identify and support youth at risk for suicide, there are gaps in building capacity and delivering program content with fidelity. A key first step in the implementation process is to determine the readiness of a school community for programming. Implementation partners should evaluate school staff and administrator attitudes toward youth suicide and perceptions of prevention. Mental health education and suicide prevention programs are typically consistent with a school's values, yet buy-in from leadership is still essential for engagement and sustained success. Leadership investment tends to drive a school's willingness to dedicate meaningful resources, including staff professional development and classroom time, messaging and family engagement, school-based mental health capacity, and collaboration with local mental health providers. Schools differ considerably with respect to resources, demographic makeup, student needs, and integration of mental healthcare. Certain districts have dedicated staff to drive comprehensive prevention and social emotional learning (SEL) efforts; in other districts, there are not a systematic approach and limited staff to support such efforts. Ideally, suicide prevention is part of a larger K–12 prevention framework with targeted interventions for students with elevated risk or mental health needs.

Assessing School Suicide Prevention Needs

Assessing school suicide prevention needs should involve a review of school and community partners, organizational capacity to deliver programming, and an exploration of barriers to adoption and sustainability. Those who plan to support suicide prevention efforts should have a clear understanding of a school community's past experiences with student suicide, attempts, and/or loss experiences by the school community. An inventory of local mental health partnerships and crisis supports with clear pathways for student support is also a prerequisite for any programming with depression and suicide screening. Awareness of cultural factors that may influence how emotional distress is expressed and to whom should be explored (see Chu et al., Chap. 11, this volume), recognizing that program adaptations and additional community engagement may be needed. Attention to historically marginalized groups and potential barriers to access of local resources are critical for planning and universal implementation (see Cwik et al., Chap. 16, this volume; Rubin et al., Chap. 13, this volume; Sheftall & Boyd, Chap. 12, this volume). Many schools have a desire to engage in suicide prevention, but implementation will often falter if there is not a strong level of guidance and collaboration around the issues noted above. External partners such as hospitals or other mental health agencies can support implementation by playing a role in convening meetings, listening to concerns, problem-solving, offsetting funding, and maintaining the momentum of school efforts.

Ensuring Sustainability

The adoption and implementation phase of a suicide prevention program is critical, but for lasting impact to be achieved, a focus on maintenance and sustainability is required. The same factors that drive success in the adoption phase may differ from those that predict success with continued delivery (Durlak & Dupre, 2008). It is common for there to be a decline in program effectiveness unless there is ongoing attention to fidelity, training, and organizational change. Problems can arise as drift from fidelity occurs and buy-in and energy around an initiative can wane. Champion turnover (i.e., the loss of a key school partner) can lead to a decline in enthusiasm, administrative capacity, and delivery skill. Diffusion of program ownership can also occur. Sustainable prevention and the institutional memory of a program should not exist in one person, or it is at high risk for failure should a role change occur. Making sure there are multiple individuals with "skin in the game" and elements of the program embedded within the school culture are key to ongoing efforts.

Several strategies exist to combat these barriers. Regular, transparent communication and two-way feedback is needed at all stages of implementation. Implementation partners should provide tools and create accessible resources for staff and students, given that school staff face many competing demands. Providing direct reinforcement, such as appreciation for their commitment, data illustrating the effectiveness of their efforts (e.g., number of youths who were identified and linked with care), and training and resources delivered at a frequency that keeps efforts top of mind without being overwhelming is ideal. Programs should seek out staff and student input regularly and incorporate changes in an iterative fashion. Family engagement should be prioritized to enhance community commitment. Program champions can be nurtured through collaborative planning meetings, continuous education, and communities of practice to learn from other schools (Flaspohler et al., 2012). Virtual trainings and consultation can enhance connection and reduce barriers for geographically isolated schools and overcome barriers posed by the recent pandemic (see Michael & Ramtekkar, Chap. 17, this volume).

Implementation in Action: Examples from Nationwide Children's Hospital

As part of an effort to expand behavioral health services in the community, Nationwide Children's Hospital (NCH) has focused on the dissemination and implementation of two universal suicide prevention programs to increase awareness, enhance early identification, and reduce youth suicide rates in the community. Throughout central and southeastern Ohio, elementary schools are offered the PAX Good Behavior Game (PAX GBG), and middle and high schools are offered an enhanced Signs of Suicide Prevention Program (SOS). These programs are offered without cost, taking a "fidelity with flexibility" approach. Both programs were selected on the basis of replicated outcome data reflecting consistent reductions in youth suicidal behaviors. PAX GBG is a universal prevention model that is implemented in schools by classroom teachers and aims to improve student self-regulation skills by promoting a nurturing school environment and prosocial student behaviors. PAX GBG targets early risk factors and fosters resiliency in elementary-aged children. Longitudinal examination shows that elementary students in PAX GBG classrooms are less likely to experience behavioral disorders, substance use, and suicidal ideation in adolescence and young adulthood (Wilcox et al., 2008).

SOS is a universal suicide prevention program delivered in middle schools and high schools that combines three critical best-practice features: (1) gatekeeper training for staff, (2) student education and guidance for seeking support, and (3) universal screening. These elements increase awareness about suicide, reduce stigma, inform students of crisis resources, and teach action steps to respond to someone displaying warning signs of suicide. SOS helps identify vulnerable students using several approaches (e.g., self-referral, standardized screening, and referral by a concerned peer/adult). In multiple RCTs, SOS has led to approximately 40–64% reductions in student self-reported suicide attempts, greater knowledge of depression and suicide, and more adaptive attitudes toward these issues (Aseltine & DeMartino, 2004; Aseltine et al., 2007; Schilling et al., 2016). These studies also find that staff display increased competence and confidence when managing at-risk students which empowers school staff to sustain this work.

Implementation of PAX GBG and Sustainability Considerations

NCH has invested in the dissemination of the PAX GBG since 2013 viewing it as a critical upstream prevention program aimed at reducing risk factors and promoting resilience. Initially, NCH primarily provided implementation and consultation support to local schools in an urban context but has since expanded efforts to include numerous rural counties. In partnership with local community agencies, including mental health boards and behavioral health agencies, the hospital supports a multi-county regional PAX GBG initiative. Three overarching research-based themes guide the hospital's approach to sustainable PAX GBG expansion:

1. Community Partnerships: The hospital sought to maximize community partnerships by including key leadership representatives from all agencies that have roles in the initiative to facilitate buy-in and shared ownership. Ongoing stakeholder meetings were held to review progress and to facilitate bidirectional feedback and continuous quality improvement efforts. Community partners took active roles in building connections with local schools and collaborators to increase local commitment to the initiative over time. Local coaches/champions (called "PAX partners") were recruited and trained to support implementation efforts in each region. Finally, a braided funding model combining local, state, and hospital funding was leveraged to expand dissemination and available consultants within the communities served.

2. Consulting: NCH took on a consulting role to support local PAX partners. These individuals were recruited and embedded in schools as a means to increase local and regional knowledge and the capacity to implement the program in the long term. Emphasis was placed on developing the expertise of local coaches through learning collaboratives, technical assistance, opportunities for PAXIS trainings, and individualized consultation.

3. Sustainability: Sustainability is discussed at the onset of partnerships with the school and local stakeholders. Sustainability plans are developed in alignment with Positive Behavioral Interventions and Supports (PBIS) and other school initiatives. A 2-year cycle of support is provided with the goal of gradually increasing local capacity to implement PAX GBG independently with the help of local coaches and school-based champions by the end of the second year.

Signs of Suicide: Scaling Up Universal Suicide Prevention with a Focus on Sustainability

The Center for Suicide Prevention and Research (CSPR) at NCH was created in 2015 to address the growing need for youth suicide prevention in Ohio with a focus on implementation of evidence-based programming and long-term viability in schools. Most schools engaged by the CSPR had never implemented a formal suicide prevention program, and other schools had embarked on time-limited efforts that ended as grants expired or as motivated partners left the table. Such outcomes demanded a different way of thinking about engagement, training, and resource utilization for suicide prevention to become a priority. Traditional approaches to program adoption have involved a partnership between a mental health organization and a school where an outside organization delivers the suicide prevention program often in collaboration with school-based mental health providers or counselors. This can result in the incomplete administration of a program or reduced levels of staff competence and effectiveness. Moreover, internal capacity to address youth suicide risk often diminishes when partnering organizations leave the building. NCH takes a different approach to training and implementation. Hospitals with a prevention focus can serve as implementation partners with an emphasis on training and practical support throughout the most challenging pieces of implementation with an eye toward independent delivery over the course of approximately 2–3 years depending on capacity and resources.

CSPR staff engage schools in an effort to build suicide prevention infrastructure in a way that addresses the unique needs of a school community. Implementation staff are licensed professional counselors and social workers with specialized training in suicide prevention, risk assessment, and safety planning. CSPR staff guide schools through two planning meetings to gauge readiness, walk through program elements, and identify school staff to support SOS implementation. Four trainings occur before SOS classroom implementation including (1) a 90-minute staff gatekeeper training to teach awareness, competence in identifying and responding to at-risk students, and confidence in using these skills, (2) a 60-minute parent/community suicide prevention gatekeeper training, (3) a 90-minute classroom presenter training to support teacher implementation of SOS curriculum and strategies for discussing suicide with youth, and (4) a 90-minute triage training to support counselors and support staff to administer and respond to positive depression/suicide screens and determine need for further risk assessment and safety planning. Following these trainings, students engage in one to two class periods of SOS program content which involves learning about depression and the risk factors and warning signs of suicide, viewing videos and discussing effective strategies to support friends displaying warning signs, and education around how to access help for yourself or a friend. This curriculum is followed by a brief depression/suicide screening. Students are also given response cards each day to request counselor support for themselves or a friend. Student screening responses are reviewed and categorized by school staff so that students with elevated suicide risk receive same-day risk assessments by onsite clinicians who obtain consent from parents/guardians and remain in communication throughout the process. Subsequently, recommendations for local services and an appropriate level of care are provided to parents. After the program is delivered, the implementation team engages in a school debriefing session held to identify opportunities for improving SOS processes. Outcomes are shared with the school and adjustments are discussed to be implemented the following year.

Sustainability is a critical goal emphasized from the first meeting. In order to build response capacity, CSPR staff provide district- or county-wide trainings in suicide risk assessment and collaborative safety planning which increase the number of community providers who are able to support school screening efforts. Local mental health partners are engaged both as referral options and as prevention partners. Initially, CSPR staff support risk assessment and safety planning on site, but providers and local mental health boards are engaged with the aim of connecting them to the schools as prevention partners to maximize sustainability. Typically, CSPR staff support is reduced by about 50% in year two, and by year three most schools can provide enhanced SOS and screening with brief consultation and planning support. The CSPR has initiated virtual communities of practice to share lessons learned and best practices in school-based suicide prevention. An evaluation of the factors that promote adoption and sustainability is a vital next step.

Policy Recommendations

1. School districts should invest in K–12 evidenced-based SEL programs that promote resiliency and reduce risk factors for suicide. Universal, suicide-specific programs should be integrated into such initiatives to maximize impact.
2. Diverse partners (such as schools, parents, youth, and mental health organizations) should be engaged to increase ownership, community buy-in, and momentum for suicide prevention efforts which is critical for successful program implementation and for driving lasting change in the school culture around mental health and suicide.
3. The implementation of school-based suicide prevention programs should incorporate a plan for sustainability throughout the prevention program cycle – from initial planning to implementation and evaluation. Tailoring the program implementation plan with school needs in mind, including training, coaching, and consultation, in collaboration with behavioral health partners is ideal.
4. Consider intentionally cultivating school-based champions to lead suicide prevention efforts, sustain them overtime, and embed programs into school culture. This effort should include robust plans for gatekeeper training, continuous education, and local communities of practice.
5. There should be investment by state and federal agencies in the development and evaluation of youth suicide prevention programs with an emphasis on fidelity with flexibility to meet the unique needs and available resources of schools with attention to prevention systems that can support sustained implementation.

Conclusion

Schools provide an important and meaningful context in which suicide prevention can occur. Schools leaders need to know not only which prevention programs work but also how to implement and sustain these programs with fidelity and flexibility to meet the needs of the community. Benefits from suicide prevention programs are fleeting when limited to a single training. Therefore, the implementation of school-based suicide prevention programs should incorporate a plan for sustainability throughout the prevention program cycle. Connecting community partners, local behavioral health organizations, and school-based champions is critical for creating lasting change. School and community cultures focused on sustainable suicide prevention can maintain gains, even after initial funding ends.

References

Aseltine, R. H., & DeMartino, R. (2004). An outcome evaluation of the SOS suicide prevention program. *American Journal of Public Health, 94*, 446–451. https://doi.org/10.2105/ajph.94.3.446

Aseltine, R. H., Jr., James, A., Schilling, E. A., & Glanovsky, J. (2007). Evaluating the SOS suicide prevention program: A replication and extension. *BMC Public Health, 7*, 161. https://doi.org/10.1186/1471-2458-7-161

Durlak, J. A., & DuPre, E. P. (2008). Implementation matters: A review of research on the influence of implementation on program outcomes and the factors affecting implementation. *American Journal of Community Psychology, 41*, 327–350. https://doi.org/10.1007/s10464-008-9165-0

Flaspohler, P. D., Meehan, C., Maras, M. A., & Keller, K. E. (2012). Ready, willing, and able: Developing a support system to promote implementation of school-based prevention programs. *American Journal of Community Psychology, 50*, 428–444. https://doi.org/10.1007/s10464-012-9520-z

Godoy Garraza, L., Kuiper, N., Goldston, D., McKean, R., & Walrath, C. (2019). Long-term impact of the Garrett Lee Smith Youth Suicide Prevention Program on youth suicide mortality, 2006–2015. *Journal of Child Psychology and Psychiatry, 60*, 1142–1147. https://doi.org/10.1111/jcpp.13058

Miller, D. N., Eckert, T. L., & Mazza, J. J. (2009). Suicide prevention programs in the schools: A review and public health perspective. *School Psychology Review, 38*, 168–188.

Nock, M. K., Green, J. G., Hwang, I., McLaughlin, K. A., Sampson, N. A., Zaslavsky, A. M., & Kessler, R. C. (2013). Prevalence, correlates, and treatment of lifetime suicidal behavior among adolescents: Results from the National Comorbidity Survey Replication Adolescent Supplement. *JAMA Psychiatry, 70*(3), 300–310. https://doi.org/10.1001/2013.jamapsychiatry.55

Schilling, E. A., Aseltine, R. H., Jr., & James, A. (2016). The SOS suicide prevention program: Further evidence of efficacy and effectiveness. *Prevention Science, 17*, 157–166. https://doi.org/10.1007/s11121-015-0594-3

Wasserman, D., Hoven, C., Wasserman, C., Wall, M., Eisenberg, R., et al. (2015). School-based suicide prevention programmes: The SEYLE cluster-randomised, controlled trial. *Lancet, 385*, 1536–1544. https://doi.org/10.1016/S0140-6736(14)61213-7

Wilcox, H. C., Kellam, S., Brown, C. H., Poduska, J., Ialongo, N., Wang, W., & Anthony, J. (2008). The impact of two universal randomized first- and second-grade classroom interventions on young adult suicide ideation and attempts. *Drug & Alcohol Dependence, 95*(Suppl 1), S60–S73.

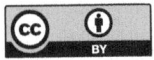

Chapter 6
Understanding Suicide Bereavement, Contagion, and the Importance of Thoughtful Postvention in Schools

Sarah Diefendorf, Sarah Van Norden, Seth Abrutyn, and Anna Mueller

Recent research estimates that one in five adolescents has been exposed to the suicide death of a family member, friend, or acquaintance during their lifetime (Andriessen et al., 2017). Understanding how youth cope with suicide loss is important since grieving early in the life course may come with unique challenges. In this review, we discuss the characteristics of adolescent suicide bereavement, research on the potential for suicide contagion, and recommended postvention practices in school settings, which can be crucial in addressing concerns about bereavement and contagion and thus help in future youth suicide prevention.

We begin by characterizing suicide loss along a continuum which contains three main categories (Cerel et al., 2014). Bereavement sits at one end of this continuum and applies to anyone who experiences long-term, significant psychological distress in response to the loss. Those affected by suicide but not bereaved may experience psychological distress, but typically less than bereaved youth. Finally, at the other end of the continuum are those who know or identify with a person who has died by suicide. The suicide loss may impact them meaningfully; however, their distress is noticeably less than those affected or bereaved. These definitions acknowledge the effects of suicide on individuals beyond the family unit, as well as variation in types of exposure and responses to suicide, and help in our understanding of appropriate assessment, support, and intervention for those who are grieving.

S. Diefendorf (✉) · A. Mueller
Department of Sociology, Indiana University Bloomington, Bloomington, IN, USA
e-mail: sdiefend@iu.edu; mueller1@iu.edu

S. Van Norden
Spatial Sciences Institute, University of Southern California, Los Angeles, CA, USA
e-mail: svannord@usc.edu

S. Abrutyn
Department of Sociology, University of British Columbia, Vancouver, BC, Canada
e-mail: sabrutyn@mail.ubc.ca

© The Author(s) 2022
J. P. Ackerman, L. M. Horowitz (eds.), *Youth Suicide Prevention and Intervention*, SpringerBriefs in Psychology,
https://doi.org/10.1007/978-3-031-06127-1_6

Suicide Bereavement

Although clinical research identifies similarities between suicide bereavement and other types of grief, suicide bereavement nevertheless has unique characteristics. Specific features of suicide loss distinguish it from death by other means, including feelings of shock, abandonment, and anger at the deceased, which may depend upon the decedent's previous history of suicidality and the perceived preventability of the suicide (Andriessen et al., 2016). Those experiencing suicide bereavement often report both physical and psychological outcomes which can include depression, PTSD, complicated (protracted) grief, and subsequent suicidality (Bottomley et al., 2019). Compared with other bereaved groups, the suicide bereaved often feel painful social emotions like responsibility, guilt, and shame (Jordan, 2001). Additionally, studies show that they are more likely to drop out of work or school and may engage in high-risk coping behaviors such as substance misuse and self-harm (Cerel & Roberts, 2005).

The context in which suicide bereavement takes place is also important. A grieving individual's social relationships, their community's shared norms, the available support systems, and the frequent stigma surrounding suicide can make suicide bereavement especially difficult (Jordan, 2001). Stigma, both external and self-imposed, can create a "double whammy" effect for the suicide bereaved who may feel simultaneously grief stricken and socially marginalized (Schreiber et al., 2017). In turn, feelings of alienation can complicate recovery. This is particularly relevant for adolescents whose grief experience intersects with a developmental stage characterized by identity formation and heightened dependency on peer relationships and perceived social acceptance (Balk, 2014).

Finally, the process of suicide bereavement and healing after suicide differs from other types of grief. Unexpected death typically elicits acute shock, but suicide often compounds this with a further need to make sense of the decedent's intentions. This can elicit a cognitive process of meaning making in which the bereaved person attempts to create a story explaining the unknown aspects of suicide, particularly why a person ended their life (Currier et al., 2015). This can prolong the mourning process, though it can also result in post-traumatic growth as individuals (a) make sense of the loss, (b) find a "silver lining" in the experience, and (c) adopt a new identity, often that of "suicide loss survivor" (Sands et al., 2011).

Adolescent Suicide Bereavement

Adolescent suicide bereavement is unique in that aspects of this developmental stage, such as identity formation, may intersect with the grieving process. Adolescence is the time of life when mental health disorders are most likely to emerge. Additionally, this is a time during which their sense of self in relation to their social world is coalescing (Balk, 2014). Adolescents tend to value peer relationships, but these relationships may become strained when an adolescent needs to process a suicide loss due to fears about stigma. Those bereaved by suicide may prefer peer support from others with similar experience in processing their grief, feeling that others who do not share their specific experience cannot appreciate their needs (Cerel et al., 2009). Informal support from peers or others with similar loss experiences may also reduce the awkwardness and stigma that can accompany suicide. However, peer support among youth raises some potential concerns; when peers support each other, they may engage in excessive and unproductive discussions of their personal challenges and mutually encourage negative talk. Such a process can increase feelings of closeness between the peers but also increase feelings of emotional distress (Andriessen et al., 2016). Peer relationships that appear outwardly supportive may mask these shared negative feelings and the peers' internalization of them, which can place adolescents at risk for adverse outcomes.

Factors That Can Impair or Facilitate Adolescent Suicide Bereavement

The mental health literacy of parents impacts how effectively parents access professional help for adolescents. Parents are often critical to getting bereaved youth professional mental health supports (Andriessen et al., 2019). When this connection is made, a trusting patient-clinician relationship is crucial for adolescents' engagement and continuation of treatment. Barriers to formal help-seeking include reliance on family, friends, or self, shame associated with mental health stigma, limited knowledge of services, and difficulty identifying symptoms of mental illness or perceiving symptoms as not meriting professional attention (Andriessen et al., 2019). Bereavement among adolescents is unique as it can leave youth vulnerable to contagion.

Social Contagion

Following a suicide, there is concern that exposure to suicide through both traditional and new media (social media and use of the internet) (Marchant et al., 2017; Ortiz & Khin Khin, 2018) or through personal role models (Abrutyn & Mueller, 2014; Maple et al., 2017; Cerel et al., 2016) puts youth at increased risk of suicidal ideation or attempt. These social influences, collectively referred to as contagion, can occur from one person to another or through a social environment, as in the case of suicide clusters or successive suicides (two or more) that occur in delimited geographic and temporal space (Haw et al., 2013; Poland et al., 2019).

Contagion research has largely focused on traditional media exposure, with recent retrospective studies suggesting that media coverage of suicides can facilitate the emergence of youth suicide clusters (Gould et al., 2014). Questions remain about how much traditional media youth consume. One recent study in Japan, for instance, found traditional media coverage following celebrity suicides was not associated with population suicide rates, though Twitter coverage was (Ueda et al., 2017). The role of social media in youth suicide is an important emerging field of research; however, studies examining the impact of exposure to suicide through social media on youth or the connection between social media and youth suicide contagion or clustering are extremely limited (Robertson et al., 2012; Ortiz & Khin Khin, 2018). One rare study of a high school suicide cluster found that youth who were posting suicide cluster-related content to their social media had a significantly higher risk of suicidal ideation (1.7 times more likely than their non-posting peers) and attempts (1.7 times) (Swedo et al., 2020); however, the study used cross-sectional data making it impossible to determine whether the observed association between posting and suicidality was because more distressed or impacted youth were more likely to post to social media or whether the posting (and ostensibly reading others' posts) generated or exacerbated youth's risk (or both). Given the importance of social media and technology to youth's lives and connections, more research is necessary to unpack the influence social media has on youth suicide bereavement as well as contagion and clustering.

Far more is known about exposure to suicide and suicide attempts through personal role models. Several decades of research using a variety of methodologies has confirmed that youth are at higher risk of suicidality after experiencing the suicide attempt or death of a friend or family member (Hawton et al., 2012; Cerel et al., 2016; Maple et al., 2017). Some hypothesize that this pattern is due to similarities in pre-existing risk factors for suicide, shared between friends or family, a phenomenon otherwise known as "homophily" or "assortative relating" (Joiner, 2007). However, multiple longitudinal studies using a variety of causal modeling strategies suggest that shared pre-existing risk factors do not fully explain this dyadic form of contagion (Baller & Richardson, 2009; Fletcher, 2017; Randall et al., 2015). In one study, researchers found that youth who had no previous suicidal history and who were exposed to a friend or family member's suicide attempt or death in the past 12 months were significantly more likely to report suicidal ideation 1 year later (Abrutyn & Mueller, 2014). Though the mechanisms through which exposure to suicide translates into increased risk of suicide are still an important area of research, studies have shown that (1) social learning, where knowledge of a friends' suicide attempt or death makes suicide more of an "option" for coping with particular forms of distress, and (2) emotional contagion contribute to suicide contagion. However, it is also worth noting that experiencing suicide loss does not always translate into increased risk of suicide; some studies show evidence of inoculation effects, where losing someone to suicide makes a person less vulnerable to suicide (Brent et al., 1993; Miklin et al., 2019). Given implications for bereaved youth, investment in additional research is justified.

Youth Suicide in Schools

Studies underscore the vulnerability of youth to suicide exposure: vulnerability that is amplified by their stage of cognitive and emotional development, which makes them especially sensitive to other's influence (Giordano, 2003). Not surprisingly, then, schools (Haw et al., 2013) and youth (Gould et al., 1989) are disproportionately susceptible to suicide clusters. Importantly, preventing suicide contagion and suicide clusters requires identifying and intervening in environmental risk factors. School contexts are important environments where youth form protective social relationships that offer youth support and meaning. However, school environments can also increase risk of suicide if they house a toxic, high-pressure culture, stigmatize mental health help-seeking, or offer few opportunities for building positive relationships with trusted adults (Mueller & Abrutyn, 2016; Pisani et al., 2012; Wyman et al., 2019). In addition, environments in which a suicide has occurred may develop a new cultural script about suicide—that is, shared beliefs about why people die by suicide, who we expect to die by suicide, and, in some cases, where, when, and how. This script can render suicide a more normative option for exposed youth, particularly if schools do not engage in adequate postvention.

School Postvention: Best Practices

Schools are critical locations for suicide postvention (see Ayer et al., this volume). While more research is needed to empirically establish the efficacy of various postvention practices, two key resources provide guidance on best practices: *After a Suicide: A Toolkit for Schools* (AFSP, 2018) and *Suicide in Schools* (Erbacher et al., 2015). These resources suggest that it is important that schools solidify a plan for postvention and establish a crisis response team long before a crisis occurs. To be effective, these plans should encompass the following four areas:

1. Community Relationships

   Schools should work to build community relationships, because while every school should have postvention practices in place, schools should never engage in postvention efforts alone. Establishing memoranda of understanding with community health officials, crisis centers, local counselors, and others who are trained in grief support and/or crisis response and can be ready to enter the school and provide extra support contributes to a more effective postvention response. Plans to draw support from the school district when possible is also advised (some districts have complementary crisis response teams). When a crisis event does occur, it is helpful to have open lines of communication with trusted community and district partners who may be able to provide extra support or interventions; for example, community partners may be able to provide trainings to school staff that highlight the typical and atypical responses in grieving and bereaved adolescents or risk factors for suicide (Erbacher et al., 2015).

2. Clear Plan of Communication

Schools should create a clear plan of communication to speak early and clearly with school staff, as well as parents and students, to help ensure that the news is delivered responsibly and sensitively (and not through informal means, like social media). Sample communications are available (see AFSP, 2018). Phone trees for staff can be useful, as can a crisis response team coordinator. Often, the first 24 hours are critical; the school should notify key personnel, while remembering that students may be hearing things before many staff due to the information flow on social media. Schools should follow guidelines for talking about suicide in all communications (AFSP, 2018, pp. 55–59). It is a school's responsibility to verify the facts of the death. Schools should be clear with all staff about what may be shared publicly (with parents) and what should not be shared. In making these decisions, it is important to respect the family's wishes regarding disclosures of details. However, if rumors are circulating among students, it may be appropriate for a trusted staff member to talk to the decedent's family and explain that talking about suicide with students can help to keep them safe (Erbacher et al., 2015).

On the first morning back at school following the loss of a student to suicide, the school should hold a meeting to provide staff with a death announcement to read to their classes. How youth hear about a death can have a profound effect on ways in which the individual responds (Hart, 2012). As such, anyone known to be very close to a deceased youth should be notified individually if possible, while the rest of the students can be told in class. The death announcement is not counseling or therapy, but a space where teachers can provide facts, dispel rumors, answer questions and normalize student reactions, and triage students following a three-tier model of crisis prevention (see Erbacher et al., 2015). Schools should also facilitate students self-referring for additional support. Staff may also be grieving and in need of support; thus, school should have substitutes or mental health professionals available to support staff.

3. Clear and Consistent Policies and Trainings

Ideally, schools will have clear and consistent policies and trainings. These policies should outline the process of recognizing and memorializing student deaths and supporting bereaved parents and impacted students and staff. School-related memorials for a suicide are a challenging issue as they can sometimes be interpreted as glorifying suicide. A standardized school policy that treats all causes of death similarly can be helpful, though this policy should be developed with all causes of death in mind to avoid stigmatizing some deaths (Gilliam, 1994; Vidal, 1989). For more details on memorializing suicide losses, we recommend reviewing *After a Suicide: A Toolkit for Schools* (AFSP, 2018, p. 60). In addition to postvention policies, strong prevention policies are also necessary. Notably, routine mental health training for school staff helps prepare staff in the event of a suicide loss. Trainings should include information on suicide and suicide myths, normalize talking about mental health and suicide, include information on cultural differences within the student body, and identify strategies to overcome potential barriers for students' access to out-of-school mental health help (e.g., language concerns, cultural beliefs about mental health, financial limitations, etc.). Trainings should address the pervasive myth that talking about suicide encourages suicide (also known as iatrogenic risk). This is not true (Joiner, 2011). This myth can be very salient during postvention as fears that a suicide may trigger contagion are common, but it is important that the community have fact-based conversations around suicide. After a suicide, such conversations are safe and necessary and likely mitigate suicide contagion.

4. Creating Space for Suicide Bereavement

Finally, schools should plan out a space within a school that, if needed, grieving students can go to, receive support, and feel safe (Erbacher et al., 2015). It is appropriate for impacted students to be invited into these spaces; however, students should be encouraged to self-refer and refer their friends as well. Scheduling meetings with vulnerable students (alone or in small groups) is another recommended approach. Collectively, these postvention strategies can help ensure a more effective suicide postvention experience.

Conclusions and Future Directions

Many youth and schools are impacted by suicide losses. Current research and practice recommendations provide sound guidance for schools to develop thoughtful postvention protocols that in turn serve as an important form of suicide *prevention*. Of course, more research is needed—particularly as new forms of communication and connection emerge—to understand the complexities of exposure to suicide during vulnerable developmental stages and to maximize the efficacy of postvention strategies. Additionally, research on suicide postvention and bereavement would benefit from a more significant emphasis on equity and strategies for postvention in contexts of resource scarcity.

References

Abrutyn, S., & Mueller, A. (2014). Are suicidal behaviors contagious? Using longitudinal data to examine suicide suggestion. *American Sociological Review, 79*(2), 211–227. https://doi.org/10.1177/0003122413519445

American Foundation for Suicide Prevention & Suicide Prevention Resource Center. (2018). *After a suicide: A toolkit for schools* (2nd ed.). Education Development Center.

Andriessen, K., Lobb, E., Mowll, J., Dudley, M., Draper, B., & Mitchell, P. B. (2019). Help-seeking experiences of bereaved adolescents: A qualitative study. *Death Studies, 43*(1), 1–8. https://doi.org/10.1080/07481187.2018.1426657

Andriessen, K., Rahman, B., Draper, B., Dudley, M., & Mitchell, P. B. (2017). Prevalence of exposure to suicide: A meta-analysis of population-based studies. *Journal of Psychiatric Research,
88*, 113–120. https://doi.org/10.1016/j.jpsychires.2017.01.017

Andriessen, K., Draper, B., Dudley, M., & Mitchell, P. B. (2016). Pre-and post-loss features of
adolescent suicide bereavement: A systematic review. *Death Studies, 40*(4), 229–246. https://
doi.org/10.1080/07481187.2015.1128497

Baller, R. & Richardson, K. (2009). The "Dark Side" of the strength of weak ties: The Diffusion
of suicidal thoughts. *Journal of Health and Social Behavior, 50*(3), 261–276. doi:https://doi.
org/10.1177/002214650905000302

Balk, D. E. (2014). *Dealing with dying, death, and grief during adolescence.* Routledge.

Bottomley, J. S., Smigelsky, M. A., Bellet, B. W., Flynn, L., Price, J., & Neimeyer, R. A. (2019).
Distinguishing the meaning making processes of survivors of suicide loss: An expansion of
the meaning of loss codebook. *Death Studies, 43*(2), 92–102. https://doi.org/10.1080/0748118
7.2018.1456011

Brent, D., Perper, J., Moritz, G., Allman, C., Friend, A., Roth, C., Schweers, J., Balach, L., &
Baugher, M. (1993). Psychiatric risk factors for adolescent suicide: A case-control study.
Journal of the American Academy of Child & Adolescent Psychiatry, 32(3), 521–529. https://
doi.org/10.1097/00004583-199305000-00006

Cerel, J., McIntosh, J. L., Neimeyer, R. A., Maple, M., & Marshall, D. (2014). The continuum of
"survivorship": Definitional issues in the aftermath of suicide. *Suicide and Life-Threatening
Behavior, 44*(6), 591–600. https://doi.org/10.1111/sltb.12093

Cerel, J., & Roberts, T. A. (2005). Suicidal behavior in the family and adolescent risk behavior.
Journal of Adolescent Health, 36(4), 352–3e8. https://doi.org/10.1016/j.jadohealth.2004.08.010

Cerel, J., Padgett, J. H., Conwell, Y., & Reed, G. A., Jr. (2009). A call for research: The need to better understand the impact of support groups for suicide survivors. *Suicide and Life-Threatening
Behavior, 39*(3), 269–281. https://doi.org/10.1521/suli.2009.39.3.269

Cerel, J., Myfanwy, M., van de Venne, J., Moore, M., Flaherty, C., & Brown, M. (2016). Exposure
to suicide in the community: Prevalence and correlates in one U.S. state. *Public Health Reports,
131*(1), 100–107. https://doi.org/10.1177/003335491613100116

Currier, J. M., Irish, J. E., Neimeyer, R. A., & Foster, J. D. (2015). Attachment, continuing bonds
and complicated grief following violent loss: Testing a moderated model. *Death Studies, 39(4),
201–210.* https://doi.org/10.1080/07481187.2014.975869

Erbacher, T. A., Singer, J. B., & Poland, S. (2015). *School-based practice in action. Suicide in
schools: A practitioner's guide to multi-level prevention, assessment, intervention, and postvention.* Routledge/Taylor & Francis Group.

Fletcher, J. M. (2017). Gender-specific pathways of peer influence on adolescent suicidal behaviors. *Socius.* https://doi.org/10.1177/2378023117729952

Gilliam, W. S. (1994, November 9–11). *Issues in student suicide prevention and sudden death
postvention: Best practices in school crisis response* [Paper presentation]. Annual Meeting of
the Mid-South Educational Research Association, Nashville, TN.

Giordano, P. C. (2003). Relationships in adolescence. *Annual Review of Sociology, 29*, 252–281.
https://doi.org/10.1146/annurev.soc.29.010202.100047

Gould, M. S., Wallenstein, S., & Davidson, L. (1989). Suicide clusters: A critical review. *Suicide
and Life-Threatening Behavior, 19*, 17–29. https://doi.org/10.1111/j.1943-278X.1989.
tb00363.x

Gould, M. S., Kleinman, M., Lake, A. M., Forman, J., & Bassett Midle, J. (2014). Newspaper
coverage of suicide and initiation of suicide clusters in teenagers in the USA, 1988–96: A
retrospective, population-based, case-control study. *Lancet Psychiatry, 1*, 34–43. https://doi.
org/10.1016/S2215-0366(14)70225-1

Haw, C., Hawton, K., Niedzwiedz, C., & Platt, S. (2013). Suicide clusters: A review
of risk factors. *Suicide and Life-Threatening Behavior, 43*(1), 97–108. https://doi.
org/10.1111/j.1943-278X.2012.00130.x

Hawton, K., Saunders, K., & O'Conner, R. C. (2012). Self-harm and suicide in adolescents. *The Lancet, 379*(9834), 2373–2382. https://doi.org/10.1016/S0140-6736(12)60322-5

Hart, J. (2012). Moving through loss: Addressing grief in our patients. *Alternative and Complementary Therapies, 18*(3), 145–147. https://doi.org/10.1089/act.2012.18301

Joiner, T. (2007). *Why people die by suicide*. Harvard University Press.

Joiner, T. (2011). *Myths about suicide*. Harvard University Press.

Jordan, J. R. (2001). Is suicide bereavement different? A reassessment of the literature. *Suicide and Life-Threatening Behavior, 31*(1), 91–102. https://doi.org/10.1521/suli.31.1.91.21310

Marchant, A., Hawton, K., Stewart, A., Montgomery, P., Singaravelu, V., Lloyd, K., Purdy, N., Daine, K., & John, A. (2017). A systematic review of the relationship between internet use, self-harm and suicidal behaviour in young people: The good, the bad and the unknown. *PloS ONE, 12*(8), e0181722. https://doi.org/10.1371/journal.pone.0181722

Miklin, S., Mueller, A. S., Abrutyn, S., & Ordonez, K. (2019). What does it mean to be exposed to suicide?: Suicide exposure, suicide risk, and the importance of meaning-making. *Social Science & Medicine, 233*(2019), 21–27. https://doi.org/10.1016/j.socscimed.2019.05.019

Mueller, A. S., & Abrutyn, S. (2016). Adolescents under pressure: A new Durkheimian framework for understanding adolescent suicide in a cohesive community. *American Sociological Review, 81*(5), 877–899. https://doi.org/10.1177/0003122416663464

Maple, M., Cerel, J., Sanford, R., Pearce, T., & Jordan, J. (2017). Is exposure to suicide beyond kin associated with risk for suicidal behavior? A systematic review of the evidence. *Suicide and Life-Threatening Behavior, 47*(4), 461–474. https://doi.org/10.1111/sltb.12308

Ortiz, P., & Khin Khin, E. (2018). Traditional and new media's influence on suicidal behavior and contagion. *Behavioral Sciences & the Law, 36*(2), 245–256. https://doi.org/10.1002/bsl.2338

Poland, S., Lieberman, R., & Niznik, M. (2019). Suicide contagion and clusters-Part 1: What school psychologists should know. *Communique, 47*(5), 21–23.

Pisani, A., Schmeelk-Cone, K., Gunzler, D., Petrova, M., Goldston, D., Tu, X., & Wyman, P. (2012). Associations between suicidal high school students' help-seeking and their attitudes and perceptions of social environment. *Journal of Youth and Adolescence, 41*, 1312–1324 https://doi.org/10.1007/s10964-012-9766-7

Randall, J. R., Nickel, N. C., & Colman, I. (2015). Contagion from peer suicidal behavior in a representative sample of American adolescents. *Journal of Affective Disorders, 186*, 219–225. https://doi.org/10.1016/j.jad.2015.07.001

Robertson, L., Skegg, K., Poore, M., Williams, S., & Taylor, B. (2012). An adolescent suicide cluster and the possible role of electronic communication technology. *Crisis, 33*(4), 239–245. https://doi.org/10.1027/0227-5910/a000140

Sands, D. C., Jordan, J. R., & Neimeyer, R. A. (2011). The meanings of suicide: A narrative approach to healing. In J. R. Jordan & J. L. McIntosh (Eds.), *Grief after suicide: Understanding the consequences and caring for the survivors* (pp. 249–282). Routledge.

Schreiber, J. K., Sands, D. C., & Jordan, J. R. (2017). The perceived experience of children bereaved by parental suicide. *OMEGA-Journal of death and dying, 75*(2), 184–206. https://doi.org/10.1177/0030222815612297

Swedo, E. A., Beauregard, J. L., de Fijter, S., Werhan, L., Norris, K., Montgomery, M. P., Rose, E. B., David-Ferdon, C., Massetti, G. M., Hillis, S. D., & Sumner, S. (2020). Associations between social media and suicidal behaviors during a youth suicide cluster in Ohio. *Journal of Adolescent Health, 68*(2), 308–316. https://doi.org/10.1016/j.jadohealth.2020.05.049

Ueda, M., Mori, K., Matsubayashi, T., & Sawada, Y. (2017). Tweeting celebrity suicides: Users' reaction to prominent suicide deaths on twitter and subsequent increases in actual suicides. *Social Science and Medicine, 189*, 158–166. https://doi.org/10.1016/j.socscimed.2017.06.032

Vidal, J. A. (1989). *Student suicide: A guide for intervention*. National Education Association.

Wyman, P., Pickering, T., Pisani, A., Rulison, K., Schmeelk-Cone, K., Hartley, M., Caine, E., LoMurray, M., Hendricks Brown, C., & Valente, T. (2019). Peer-adult network structure and suicide attempts in 38 high schools: implications for network-informed suicide prevention. *The Journal of Child Psychology and Psychiatry, 60*(10), 1065–1075. https://doi.org/10.1111/jcpp.13102

Part III
Suicide-Specific Intervention

Chapter 7
Utilizing Suicide Risk Screening as a Prevention Technique in Pediatric Medical Settings

Annabelle M. Mournet, Nathan J. Lowry, and Lisa M. Horowitz

Pediatricians and other medical providers are de facto mental health providers on the front lines of the public health crisis of youth suicide and are uniquely positioned to recognize warning signs and help young people develop effective coping strategies for managing emotional distress (Kessler & Stafford, 2008). Universal screening for suicide risk, which involves screening all patients regardless of presenting problem, in all medical settings, including primary care, is supported and encouraged by many organizations, including the American Academy of Pediatrics (AAP), The Joint Commission (TJC), and the National Action Alliance for Suicide Prevention (NAASP) (Shain & Committee on Adolescence, 2016; TJC, 2016; NAASP, 2012). Implementing suicide risk screening and assessment with evidence-based tools can enhance feasibility of screening for suicide risk without overburdening busy systems of care (Horowitz et al., 2010, 2020). Moreover, screening has been identified as an effective suicide prevention tool (NAASP, 2012). Through education and training, pediatric providers can be pivotal partners in detecting suicide risk and connecting their patients to mental health treatments. This chapter will highlight how utilizing evidence-based screening tools and clinical pathways to manage patients that screen positive can be feasible and potentially lifesaving.

Medical Settings as Venues for Suicide Risk Screening

Medical settings are uniquely positioned to screen for suicide risk as they are a major point of connection between trusted adults and youth. From a public health perspective, the majority of youth in the USA have annual contact with physicians

A. M. Mournet · N. J. Lowry · L. M. Horowitz (✉)
Office of the Clinical Director, National Institute of Mental Health, Bethesda, MD, USA
e-mail: nathan.lowry@nih.gov; horowitzl@mail.nih.gov

© The Author(s) 2022
J. P. Ackerman, L. M. Horowitz (eds.), *Youth Suicide Prevention and Intervention*, SpringerBriefs in Psychology,
https://doi.org/10.1007/978-3-031-06127-1_7

in emergency departments (EDs), hospitals, and outpatient primary care settings. Youth are also typically accompanied to healthcare settings by parents or caregivers which is crucial for effective assessment, intervention, and safety planning. Of note, death registry studies show that 80% of adolescents who die by suicide visited a healthcare setting in the months or even weeks prior to their death (Ahmedani et al., 2014; Rhodes et al., 2013), whereas only 20% of suicide decedents had contact with a mental health professional in the month prior to their death by suicide (Luoma et al., 2002). For some, nonbehavioral health venues may be the only healthcare contact where an individual's suicide risk can be identified.

In an effort to reduce youth suicide rates, which have increased steadily over the past decade (see Ruch & Bridge, Chap. 1, this volume), TJC has highlighted medical settings as critical venues for suicide risk detection by issuing Sentinel Event Alert 56 (SEA 56), urging medical settings to screen all medical patients for suicide risk using brief, evidence-based screening tools (TJC, 2016). TJC also updated National Patient Safety Goal 15 (NPSG 15) in 2019 to enhance patient safety and healthcare delivery for both behavioral health patients and medical patients at risk for suicide (TJC, 2019). As a result of SEA 56 and NPSG 15, many medical settings have begun implementing suicide risk screening, further necessitating validated suicide risk screening tools for use among medical patients. Numerous institutions have already reported on their considerable progress implementing screening among pediatric medical patients (Roaten et al., 2021; Lois et al., 2020). The experiences of these institutions have demonstrated that obtaining stakeholder endorsement, establishing a dedicated interdisciplinary work group, and appropriately managing positive screens are essential to a screening program's sustainability (Roaten et al., 2021; Snyder et al., 2020). There are also gaps in understanding and executing effective screening programs; please see TJC website for guidance (https://www.jointcommission.org/resources/patient-safety-topics/suicide-prevention/). Medical patients typically present with somatic chief complaints and rarely disclose suicidal thoughts unless directly asked (Pan et al., 2009), requiring systematic suicide risk screening of medical patients to detect suicide risk that would otherwise go undetected. It is important to use tools that are evidence-based and, when possible, created for the targeted age group and validated in the settings in which they are going to be used. A review by Thom et al. (2020) highlighted several well-validated suicide risk screening tools for use in medical settings, including the Ask Suicide-Screening Questions (ASQ; Horowitz et al., 2012) and the Patient Safety Screener (PSS; Boudreaux et al., 2015), that were designed for and validated among medical patients (Thom et al., 2020). Additionally, new tools continue to be developed, such as the Computerized Adaptive Screen for Suicidal Youth (CASSY; King et al., 2021), which take advantage of new technologies to enhance screening processes in the ED.

Barriers to Address

Prior to implementing a suicide risk screening program, several barriers may need to be addressed. First, there is a common myth that asking someone questions about suicide can "put ideas in their head" and cause someone to have thoughts of suicide. This myth may lead providers and families to have concerns about or avoid suicide risk screening. However, this potential iatrogenic risk of screening has been refuted in multiple studies (Gould et al., 2005; DeCou & Schumann, 2018). In fact, one of the most effective ways to keep a young person from killing themselves is by asking them directly, "Are you thinking of killing yourself?", and then listening empathetically, and responding supportively.

Suicide Risk Screening Clinical Pathways

Often, healthcare providers recognize the need for suicide risk identification but feel ill-equipped to build screening into routine practice. To provide physicians with step-by-step instructions on how to manage patients at risk for suicide and to address some of the barriers surrounding suicide risk screening, the American Academy of Child and Adolescent Psychiatry (AACAP) sponsored the creation of youth suicide risk screening clinical pathways (Brahmbhatt et al., 2019). These screening pathways were designed to allow each medical facility the flexibility to adapt screening procedures based on available staff and resources. The pathways use a three-tiered system that begins with a nurse/medical assistant administering the ASQ as a brief screen. Next, if a patient screens positive for suicide risk, a mental health clinician, nurse practitioner, physician assistant, or physician conducts a Brief Suicide Safety Assessment (BSSA) using the Columbia-Suicide Severity Rating Scale (C-SSRS; Posner et al., 2011) or the ASQ Brief Suicide Safety Assessment (ASQ BSSA; NIMH, 2017). The second step of the pathway, administering a BSSA, is critical as it aides the clinician in quickly determining next steps for a patient who screens positive for suicide risk. Finally, the third step of the clinical pathway utilizes the risk assessment results to determine whether the patient proceeds to a full mental health evaluation, a mental health referral, or safety planning and resources. The pathways were designed to be flexible and adaptable to each venue's institutional milieu and can be adapted in a way that was most functional for the institution implementing the tools.

Suicide risk screening of medical patients may be especially challenging when in-person visits are restricted such as during the COVID-19 pandemic. Although data are not yet available regarding how the recent pandemic affected the overall youth suicide rate, there remains an urgent need to continue screening for suicide risk. To address this need, COVID-19 suicide risk screening clinical pathways were developed to guide clinicians through screening for suicide risk via telehealth/phone to effectively manage patients who screen positive (Pao et al., 2020). Typically, individuals with acute suicidal thoughts require an urgent psychiatric evaluation in an ED. The pathway was revised to help patients at acute suicide risk and their parents/guardians find alternatives to going to the ED in order to avoid exposure to COVID-19 and also spare the ED from over-crowding during the pandemic. In addition to the over-crowding problems created for the healthcare system, unnecessary ED visit can be traumatizing and costly to families (Lerwick, 2016), and therefore is not an effective intervention. A critical part of this pathway is for the healthcare practitioner to provide lethal means safety counseling (see Monahan & Stanley, Chap. 9, this volume) to the patient and family members or friends to ensure safe storage or removal of potentially dangerous items (e.g., pills, firearms, belts, knives). Separate adult and youth versions of this pathway were created and are available as part of the ASQ Toolkit (www.nih.nimh/ASQ).

Feasibility of Screening

Screening for suicide risk has been shown to be feasible in both large and small healthcare systems (Roaten et al., 2021; Snyder et al., 2020; Tipton et al., 2019). In order to successfully implement a screening program, it is important to enact quality improvement processes, such as a Plan-Do-Study-Act quality improvement (QI) framework (Deming, 1993). The iterative QI framework aims to raise the standard of care for all patients and begins with formalizing a plan for what the elevated standard of care should be, followed by training and education to achieve this standard. A pilot phase in which individuals can provide suggestions for improvement allows for continuous improvements to be made as research advances. Using a QI approach, suicide risk screening was successfully implemented at a suburban pediatric primary care practice in Richmond, Virginia (Tipton et al., 2019). Following the iterative Plan-Do-Study-Act QI approach, medical staff were trained to administer screening and to manage patients who screened positive for suicide risk. During this process, unanticipated problems were identified and addressed. For example, upon receiving numerous questions from parents, an informational flyer for parents was circulated at the clinic to announce the new addition of suicide risk screening to standard practice. By using a QI methodology, suicide risk screening was successfully implemented with both nurses and physicians who indicated that screening did not disrupt clinic workflow and that they felt comfortable screening and managing patients for suicide risk (Tipton et al., 2019). The ASQ tool is available publicly in the ASQ Toolkit in many different languages (www.nih.nimh/ASQ). Resources for other commonly used screeners, like the C-SSRS, are available (www.cssrs.columbia.edu).

Screening Underserved Populations

Black, Indigenous, and people of color (BIPOC) youth have been historically excluded in suicide research. When universally screening for suicide risk, it is important to use screening tools that are valid for use among groups at higher risk. Similarly, screening tools need to be culturally and psychometrically sensitive. The ASQ has been translated into 18 languages, but to maintain its psychometric properties, there was a need to go beyond verbatim translation. For example, the ASQ tool was considered for use in a medical facility that served members of the Navajo Nation. There were concerns about how screening would be perceived, as the ASQ has items that ask directly about suicide using words like "death," which is a taboo word in this culture. Changing the language of validated tools is typically advised against; however, measures are often validated in contexts that do not account for cultural differences, and administering to a new group without accounting for these factors may be equally problematic. With input from members of the Navajo Nation, researchers created a Diné version of the ASQ specifically for members of the Navajo Nation which replaced the word "death" with "not alive." Whenever changing the language of a tool, it is important to retest it. A study is underway to validate this version of the tool to ensure that it still accurately identifies suicide risk. Linguistic differences should also be considered when translating suicide risk screening tools.

Conclusion

Medical settings represent one of the few opportunities for young people to disclose mental health issues and be connected to resources. Through implementing QI methodology and using three-tiered suicide risk screening clinical pathways, evidence-based suicide risk screening programs are achievable and can allow healthcare systems to feasibly integrate screening into practice. To ensure that universal suicide risk screening programs are truly "universal," we must question whether our tools and pathways work for all intended populations. Specifically, providers should evaluate whether screening instruments and assessment approaches are effective for understudied populations who may also be at high risk for suicide. Providers should also consider how they gather and act on feedback from communities as well as individuals with lived experience (see Rowan et al., Chap. 18, this volume). Future research, clinical practices, and policies must focus on addressing the needs of high-risk populations to ensure screening tools accurately identify risk among all individuals and are culturally sensitive.

Acknowledgments The authors would like to thank Patrick Ryan for his assistance in preparing this chapter.

Funding Details This research was supported in part by the Intramural Research Program of the NIMH (Annual Report Number ZIAMH002922).

References

Ahmedani, B. K., Simon, G. E., Stewart, C., Beck, A., Waitzfelder, B. E., Rossom, R., Lynch, F., Owen-Smith, A., Hunkeler, E. M., Whiteside, U., Operskalski, B. H., Coffey, M. J., & Solberg, L. I. (2014). Health care contacts in the year before suicide death. *Journal of General Internal Medicine, 29*(6), 870–877. https://doi.org/10.1007/s11606-014-2767-3

Boudreaux, E. D., Jaques, M. L., Brady, K. M., Matson, A., & Allen, M. H. (2015). The patient safety screener: Validation of a brief suicide risk screener for emergency department settings. *Archives of Suicide Research, 19*(2), 151–160. https://doi.org/10.1080/13811118.2015.1034604

Brahmbhatt, K., Kurtz, B. P., Afzal, K. I., Giles, L. L., Kowal, E. D., Johnson, K. P., Lanzillo, E., Pao, M., Plioplys, S., Horowitz, L. M., & PaCC Workgroup. (2019). Suicide risk screening in pediatric hospitals: Clinical pathways to address a global health crisis. *Psychosomatics, 60*(1), 1–9. https://doi.org/10.1016/j.psym.2018.09.003

DeCou, C. R., & Schumann, M. E. (2018). On the iatrogenic risk of assessing suicidality: A meta-analysis. *Suicide & Life-Threatening Behavior, 48*(5), 531–543. https://doi.org/10.1111/sltb.12368

Deming, W. E. (1993). *The new economics for industry, government, education.* Massachusetts Institute of Technology, Center for Advanced Engineering Study.

Gould, M. S., Marrocco, F. A., Kleinman, M., Thomas, J. G., Mostkoff, K., Cote, J., & Davies, M. (2005). Evaluating iatrogenic risk of youth suicide screening programs: A randomized controlled trial. *JAMA, 293*(13), 1635–1643. https://doi.org/10.1001/jama.293.13.1635

Horowitz, L., Ballard, E., Teach, S. J., Bosk, A., Rosenstein, D. L., Joshi, P., Dalton, M. E., & Pao, M. (2010). Feasibility of screening patients with nonpsychiatric complaints for suicide risk in a pediatric emergency department: A good time to talk? *Pediatric Emergency Care, 26*(11), 787–792. https://doi.org/10.1097/PEC.0b013e3181fa8568

Horowitz, L. M., Bridge, J. A., Teach, S. J., Ballard, E., Klima, J., Rosenstein, D. L., Wharff, E. A., Ginnis, K., Cannon, E., Joshi, P., & Pao, M. (2012). Ask Suicide-Screening Questions (ASQ): A brief instrument for the pediatric emergency department. *Archives of Pediatrics & Adolescent Medicine, 166*(12), 1170–1176. https://doi.org/10.1001/archpediatrics.2012.1276

Horowitz, L. M., Wharff, E. A., Mournet, A. M., Ross, A. M., McBee-Strayer, S., He, J. P., Lanzillo, E.vC., White, E., Bergdoll, E., Powell, D. S., Solages, M., Merikangas, K. R., Pao, M., & Bridge, J. A. (2020). Validation and feasibility of the ASQ among pediatric medical and surgical inpatients. *Hospital Pediatrics, 10*(9), 750–757. https://doi.org/10.1542/hpeds.2020-0087

Kessler, R., & Stafford, D. (2008). Primary care is the De Facto mental health system. In R. Kessler & D. Stafford (Eds.), *Collaborative medicine case studies.* Springer. https://doi.org/10.1007/978-0-387-76894-6_2

King, C. A., Brent, D., Grupp-Phelan, J., Casper, T. C., Dean, J. M., Chernick, L. S., Fein, J. A., Mahabee-Gittens, E. M., Patel, S. J., Mistry, R. D., Duffy, S., Melzer-Lange, M., Rogers, A., Cohen, D. M., Keller, A., Shenoi, R., Hickey, R. W., Rea, M., Cwik, M., ... Pediatric Emergency Care Applied Research Network. (2021). Prospective development and validation of the computerized adaptive screen for suicidal youth. *JAMA Psychiatry, 78*(5), 540–549. https://doi.org/10.1001/jamapsychiatry.2020.4576

Lerwick, J. L. (2016). Minimizing pediatric healthcare-induced anxiety and trauma. *World Journal of Clinical Pediatrics, 5*(2), 143–150. https://doi.org/10.5409/wjcp.v5.i2.143

Lois, B. H., Urban, T. H., Wong, C., Collins, E., Brodzinsky, L., Harris, M. A., Adkisson, H., Armstrong, M., Pontieri, J., Delgado, D., Levine, J., & Liaw, K. R. (2020). Integrating suicide risk screening into pediatric ambulatory subspecialty care. *Pediatric Quality & Safety, 5*(3), e310. https://doi.org/10.1097/pq9.0000000000000310

Luoma, J. B., Martin, C. E., & Pearson, J. L. (2002). Contact with mental health and primary care providers before suicide: A review of the evidence. *The American Journal of Psychiatry, 159*(6), 909–916. https://doi.org/10.1176/appi.ajp.159.6.909

National Action Alliance for Suicide Prevention. (2012). *2012 national strategy for suicide prevention: Goals and objectives for action: A report of the U.S. Surgeon General and of the National Action Alliance for suicide prevention*. US Department of Health & Human Services.

National Institute of Mental Health. (2017). *ASQ suicide risk screening toolkit. Screening youth for suicide risk in medical settings*. Available at: www.nimh.nih.gov/ASQ

Pan, Y. J., Lee, M. B., Chiang, H. C., & Liao, S. C. (2009). The recognition of diagnosable psychiatric disorders in suicide cases' last medical contacts. *General Hospital Psychiatry, 31*(2), 181–184. https://doi.org/10.1016/j.genhosppsych.2008.12.010

Pao, M., Mournet, A. M., & Horowitz, L. M. (2020). Implementation challenges of universal suicide risk screening in adult patients in general medical and surgical settings. *Psychiatric Times, 37*(7), 25–27.

Posner, K., Brown, G. K., Stanley, B., Brent, D. A., Yershova, K. V., Oquendo, M. A., Currier, G. W., Melvin, G. A., Greenhill, L., Shen, S., & Mann, J. J. (2011). The Columbia-Suicide Severity Rating Scale: Initial validity and internal consistency findings from three multisite studies with adolescents and adults. *The American Journal of Psychiatry, 168*(12), 1266–1277. https://doi.org/10.1176/appi.ajp.2011.10111704

Rhodes, A. E., Khan, S., Boyle, M. H., Tonmyr, L., Wekerle, C., Goodman, D., Bethell, J., Leslie, B., Lu, H., & Manion, I. (2013). Sex differences in suicides among children and youth: The potential impact of help-seeking behaviour. *Canadian Journal of Psychiatry, 58*(5), 274–282. https://doi.org/10.1177/070674371305800504

Roaten, K., Horowitz, L. M., Bridge, J. A., Goans, C., McKintosh, C., Genzel, R., Johnson, C., & North, C. S. (2021). Universal pediatric suicide risk screening in a health care system: 90,000 patient encounters. *Journal of the Academy of Consultation-Liaison Psychiatry, 62*(4), 421–429. https://doi.org/10.1016/j.jaclp.2020.12.002

Shain, B., & Committee on Adolescence (2016). Suicide and suicide attempts in adolescents. *Pediatrics, 138*(1), e20161420. https://doi.org/10.1542/peds.2016-1420

Snyder, D. J., Jordan, B. A., Aizvera, J., Innis, M., Mayberry, H., Raju, M., Lawrence, D., Dufek, A., Pao, M., & Horowitz, L. M. (2020). From pilot to practice: Implementation of a suicide risk screening program in hospitalized medical patients. *Joint Commission Journal on Quality and Patient Safety, 46*(7), 417–426. https://doi.org/10.1016/j.jcjq.2020.04.011

The Joint Commission. (2016). Detecting and treating suicide ideation in all settings. *Sentinel Event Alert Issue, 56*(56), 1–7.

The Joint Commission. (2019). *National Patient Safety Goal 15.01.01 R3 Report*. www.jointcommission.org/-/media/tjc/documents/standards/r3-reports/r3_18_suicide_prevention_hap_bhc_cah_11_4_19_final1.pdf. Accessed 17 Feb 2021.

Thom, R., Hogan, C., & Hazen, E. (2020). Suicide risk screening in the hospital setting: A review of brief validated tools. *Psychosomatics, 61*(1), 1–7. https://doi.org/10.1016/j.psym.2019.08.009

Tipton, M. V., Abernathy, T., Lanzillo, E. C., Powell, D., Snyder, D., Bridge, J., Schoenbaum, M., Pao, M., & Horowitz, L. M. (2019). 1.67 Implementing suicide risk screening in pediatric primary care: From research to practice. *Journal of the American Academy of Child & Adolescent Psychiatry, 58*(10).

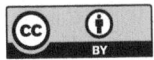

Chapter 8
After Screening: A Developmentally Informed Approach to Safety Planning and Stabilization

Lucas Zullo, Tamar Kodish, and Joan Asarnow

This chapter focuses on clinical interventions after a youth has been evaluated as showing signs of suicide risk. We build on evidence-based approaches for identifying youth at risk for suicide (see Mournet et al., Chap. 7, this volume) and focus on Safe Alternatives for Teens and Youths-Acute (SAFETY-A, also known as the Family Intervention for Suicide Prevention, FISP), a brief therapeutic assessment and intervention that emphasizes stability, safety, and linkage. This approach has potential for preventing unnecessary and costly hospitalizations, which have variable effectiveness compared to intensive community-based outpatient services (Giles et al., 2021; Hutcherson et al., 2021; Coyle et al., 2018; Hughes et al., 2017). Such brief interventions aim to elicit behaviors and protective factors that mitigate the risk of suicidal behavior and allow for transition to outpatient care for youth who might otherwise require extended hospitalization or acute behavioral healthcare to maintain safety.

State of the Evidence: What Have We Learned?

Currently, there are several interventions that have shown promise for reducing suicide attempts and suicide attempt risk in randomized controlled trials (RCTs) with youth. Three interventions have shown efficacy for reducing suicide attempts in single RCTs relative to comparison conditions: Integrated Cognitive Behavior Therapy for Suicidality and Substance Abuse (Esposito-Smythers et al., 2011); the 12-week SAFETY treatment, a DBT-informed cognitive behavioral and family

L. Zullo (✉) · T. Kodish · J. Asarnow
Department of Psychiatry and Biobehavioral Sciences, University of California, Los Angeles, CA, USA
e-mail: LZullo@mednet.ucla.edu; tamarkodish@ucla.edu; jasarnow@mednet.ucla.edu

© The Author(s) 2022
J. P. Ackerman, L. M. Horowitz (eds.), *Youth Suicide Prevention and Intervention*, SpringerBriefs in Psychology,
https://doi.org/10.1007/978-3-031-06127-1_8

treatment (Asarnow et al., 2017); and Dialectical Behavior Therapy (DBT, McCauley et al., 2018). DBT has also been classified as a "well-established" intervention for self-harm, inclusive of both suicidal and non-suicidal self-injurious behavior, based on evidence from three independent RCTs (Mehlum et al., 2019; McCauley et al., 2018; Santamarina-Perez et al., 2020). Five "probably efficacious" interventions for self-injurious thoughts and behaviors have also been identified. These include cognitive behavioral therapy with individual and family components, interpersonal therapy for adolescents, psychodynamic therapy with individual and family components, integrated family therapy, and parent training (for review, see Glenn et al., 2019). Additional promising suicide-specific interventions include attachment-based family therapy (Diamond et al., 2010), as well as Cognitive Behavioral Therapy for Suicide Prevention (CBT-SP) (Stanley et al., 2009) and the Collaborative Assessment and Management of Suicidality (CAMS) (Jobes et al., 2019), both of which have been tested primarily in adults. Because successful replication of benefits for reducing self-harm in youth was identified only for DBT, and there have been failures to replicate benefits, continued research to replicate and extend these findings is needed. Research is also needed to test interventions among youth from diverse backgrounds (e.g., racial and ethnic minority youth, LGBTQ+ youth, urban vs. rural, youth in foster care) to determine the degree to which treatment benefits extend to heterogeneous groups of youth presenting with suicide and self-harm risk.

Despite emerging data pointing to effective treatments for suicidality and self-harm, the majority of youth at risk for suicide do not receive care, and racial/ethnic minority youth are less likely to receive evidence-based treatments (EBTs) relative to nonminority youth (Wu et al., 2010; Asarnow & Miranda, 2014). Racial and ethnic minority youth may be particularly likely to benefit from EBTs (Ngo et al., 2009; Adrian et al., 2019), underscoring the value that integrating evidence-based suicide prevention into community care may have in reducing racial disparities in mental health. To accomplish this goal, barriers such as systematic racism and structural inequity within our healthcare systems must be addressed through policy initiatives. In addition, interventions designed to enhance continuity of care for suicidal youth should be implemented in routine care settings, and strategies that support sustainability of these programs are needed.

SAFETY-A

In this section, we illustrate one promising suicide-specific care model used with adolescents with initial evidence of effectiveness. SAFETY-A is a therapeutic assessment approach which aims to achieve three primary aims: (1) provide crisis intervention for youth presenting with suicidal episodes; (2) enhance youth safety; and (3) improve linkage to follow-up care and continuity of care. Results of a two-site RCT indicate that SAFETY-A is effective in improving rates of linkage to follow-up treatment after an emergency department (ED) visit for suicidal ideation or behavior (Asarnow et al., 2011). This is an important outcome and treatment goal, as rates of follow-up treatment are low in this population and receiving follow-up care is a necessary condition for receiving effective treatment. Of note, improving continuity of care is listed as Objective 8.4 of our National Strategy for Suicide Prevention (United States Department of Health and Human Services, 2012).

Figure 8.1 illustrates how SAFETY-A fits into a care process model for treating youth presenting with elevated risk for suicide. Following initial identification of suicide or self-harm risk, and medical clearance, SAFETY-A provides additional evaluation and brief therapeutic intervention. Initially developed for use in the ED and based on an earlier specialized ED intervention (Rotheram-Borus et al., 1996), SAFETY-A can be completed in 20–90 minutes depending on available time, allowing for adjustments based on youth and parent/caregiver response and practical considerations (Asarnow et al., 2009, 2020).

This strengths-based, developmentally nuanced approach includes five key youth tasks and three parent/caregiver (hereafter referred to as parents) tasks. These "tasks" aim to assess whether the clinician can elicit behaviors that are incompatible with suicidal thoughts and self-harm. Youth tasks include (1) identifying three strengths in the youth and family/environment; (2) understanding the youth's emotional reactions using an "emotional thermometer"; (3) participating in safety planning in which the youth identifies skills/strategies that can be used instead of self-harm; (4) identifying a minimum of three people the youth can go to for support in staying safe (emphasizing responsible adults); and (5) making a commitment to using the safety plan instead of resorting to self-harm behavior. The clinician also provides some counseling on means restriction and the potential disinhibiting effects of substance use.

By leading with a focus on strengths, a clinician disrupts the emphasis on problem behavior and provides an opportunity for the youth to focus on content that is associated with feelings of self-worth, hopeful thoughts, and reasons for living.

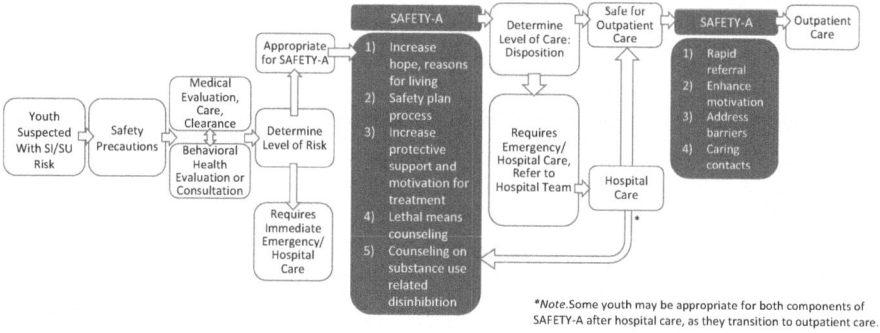

Note. Some youth may be appropriate for both components of SAFETY-A after hospital care, as they transition to outpatient care.

© Joan R Asarnow, PhD

Fig. 8.1 SAFETY-A care process model

Changing the tone of crisis care in this way allows the clinician to build rapport with the youth, shift the focus to thoughts and behaviors that are incompatible with suicide/suicide attempts, and gather key information that can be used in safety planning. Conversely, if a youth is unable to identify strengths in themselves or the environment, this may be an indicator that additional evaluation and intensive support is needed prior to discharge to home or a lower level of care.

Parent tasks feature the following elements: (1) identifying three strengths in the youth and family/environment; (2) committing to and developing a plan for restricting access to dangerous self-harm methods (e.g., firearms) and increasing supportive monitoring and protective supervision; and (3) enhancing caregiver ability to support youth in using the safety plan instead of self-harm. When a parent is unavailable, parent involvement is contraindicated (e.g., abuse), and/or there are other key caregivers; this work can also include or substitute significant others in the youth's life. Safety planning should attend to the youth's current social environment (e.g., outreach to noncustodial parent and adults with whom the youth may reside).

Several promising findings have emerged using this model. After an average of 2 months, youth receiving SAFETY-A were significantly more likely to attend outpatient treatment; receive psychotherapy; and had more psychotherapy visits. However, analyses (adjusting for selection biases in receipt of treatment) did not result in benefits of linkage to community treatment as usual (Asarnow et al., 2011). While this trial did not indicate SAFETY-A led to improved clinical outcomes, the assessment approximately 2 months after hospital discharge may have been too late to detect clinical response. This is suggested by results from the earlier/first-generation ED intervention which indicated decreased suicidal ideation at an immediate post-discharge evaluation (Rotheram-Borus et al., 1996). In addition, open trial data of response to SAFETY-A in an outpatient crisis clinic indicated that after delivery of SAFETY-A, youth and parents reported significant improvements in their confidence that they could keep themselves or their children safe (Zullo et al., 2020). Significant reductions were also seen from pre- to post-intervention in youths' urges to self-harm, intent to end their lives by suicide, and level of misery/unhappiness.

Importantly, both an earlier trial with the early/first-generation version of SAFETY-A and a later trial that incorporated the emergency/SAFETY-A intervention as the first session of a more extended yet still brief follow-up treatment found reduced suicidality relative to comparison conditions (Rotheram-Borus et al., 2000; Asarnow et al., 2017). These studies support the benefits of the SAFETY-A approach for reducing suicide attempt risk when combined with a suicide-focused evidence-informed intervention. Specifically, the data support SAFETY-A is an effective first step during the transition to evidence-based programs such as DBT or longer-term treatments such as SAFETY or Integrated CBT. Moreover, SAFETY-A has some key overlap with longer-term treatments and sets the groundwork for an initial follow-up session by establishing safety through the creation of a developmentally informed safety plan. SAFETY-A complements these evidence-based modalities by targeting the critical component of safety before follow-up care is administered. Typical recommended courses of action following SAFETY-A are supporting the rapid linkage to evidence-based care and protective action from caregivers as needed during this transition period.

Conclusions and Policy Implications

It is critical that healthcare settings offer evidence-based suicide-specific interventions to youth at risk for suicide. In addition to outpatient treatment modalities such as DBT, CBT-SP, CAMS, and other interpersonal, dynamic, and cognitive behavioral treatments with support, brief targeted emergency department intervention can have a positive impact. SAFETY-A fills a critical gap in the clinical pathway for treating suicidal youth (Fig. 8.1). After a youth screens positive for elevated suicide risk, a brief therapeutic intervention to further assess risk and enhance safety for youth who can be safely discharged home is an important next step. Use of SAFETY-A to further assess risk and offer a brief intervention allows for improved access to evidence-based suicide prevention care, with the potential for especially large benefits for racial and ethnic minority youth who often lack access to such care (Asarnow & Miranda, 2014).

Suicide-specific care models have the potential to drive improved intervention outcomes among vulnerable youth. We highlighted how one such evidence-based approach, SAFETY-A, contributes to enhanced evaluation, safety planning, and linkage after a positive screen for suicide risk. SAFETY-A represents a critical next step as screening without effective therapeutic intervention may contribute to poor outcomes (e.g., elevated readmission and suicide rates) and increase burden on the healthcare system and families. Early results suggest integrated mental health and medical care can help reduce the financial burden of mental health problems emerging after a suicide loss (Perrin et al., 2019). Now that strong evidence-based approaches to screening have been developed (Mournet et al., Chap. 7, this volume), research and quality improvement efforts should consider how to best augment screening by increasing the availability of effective therapeutic assessments and follow-up care.

One such initiative to increase access to evidence-based care for youth suicide prevention is through the UCLA-Duke Center for Trauma-Informed Suicide, Self-Harm & Substance Abuse Treatment & Prevention ASAP Center (SAMHSA U79SM08004). Given the strong association between suicide/self-harm risk and trauma exposure, the ASAP Center advances the dissemination and implementation of evidence-based interventions for youth mental health by offering resources and trainings on trauma-informed care, SAFETY-A, and the 12-week SAFETY program and integrating effective strategies for evaluating and reducing suicide and self-harm risk in primary care, emergency, school, and other key service settings (Goldston & Asarnow, 2021). More information on the ASAP Center resources and programs can be found at https://asapnctsn.org/.

SAFETY-A and other promising suicide-specific intervention approaches have the potential to increase the chances that youth at risk for suicide receive care that

meets their individual needs for safety, stability, family support, and ongoing therapeutic care. Ultimately, this type of work is highly complementary of existing suicide prevention efforts. It is our hope that clinicians and policy makers will use this
information to enhance suicide care in their communities and prevent premature
deaths and suffering among our youth.

Funding Details   Dr. Asarnow has received grant, research, or other support from the National
Institute of Mental Health, the American Foundation for Suicide Prevention, the Substance Abuse
and Mental Health Services Administration, the American Psychological Association (APA), the
Society of Clinical Child and Adolescent Psychology (Division 53 of the APA), the American
Psychological Foundation, and the Association for Child and Adolescent Mental Health. She has
served as a consultant on quality improvement for depression and suicide/self-harm prevention and
serves on the Scientific Council of the American Foundation for Suicide Prevention and the
Scientific Advisory Board of the Klingenstein Third Generation Foundation. Work on this chapter
was supported partly by National Institutes of Health under Award Number R01MH112147-04S1.
The content is solely the responsibility of the authors and does not necessarily represent the official
views of the National Institutes of Health.

References

Adrian, M., McCauley, E., Berk, M. S., Asarnow, J. R., Korslund, K., Avina, C., Gallop, R., &
Linehan, M. M. (2019). Predictors and moderators of recurring self-harm in adolescents participating in a comparative treatment trial of psychological interventions. *Journal of Child
Psychology and Psychiatry, and Allied Disciplines, 60*(10), 1123–1132. https://doi.org/10.1111/
jcpp.13099

Asarnow, J. R., & Miranda, J. (2014). Improving care for depression and suicide risk in adolescents: Innovative strategies for bringing treatments to community settings. *Annual Review of
Clinical Psychology, 10*, 275–303. https://doi.org/10.1146/annurev-clinpsy-032813-153742

Asarnow, J. R., Berk, M. S., & Baraff, L. J. (2009). Family intervention for suicide prevention: A
specialized emergency department intervention for suicidal youths. *Professional Psychology:
Research and Practice, 40*(2), 118. https://doi.org/10.1037/a0012599

Asarnow, J. R., Baraff, L. J., Berk, M., Grob, C. S., Devich-Navarro, M., Suddath, R., Piacentini,
J. C., Rotheram-Borus, M. J., Cohen, D., & Tang, L. (2011). An emergency department
intervention for linking pediatric suicidal patients to follow-up mental health treatment.
Psychiatric Services (Washington, DC), 62(11), 1303–1309. https://doi.org/10.1176/ps.62.11.
pss6211_1303

Asarnow, J. R., Hughes, J. L., Babeva, K. N., & Sugar, C. A. (2017). Cognitive-behavioral
family treatment for suicide attempt prevention: A randomized controlled trial. *Journal
of the American Academy of Child & Adolescent Psychiatry, 56*(6), 506–514. https://doi.
org/10.1016/j.jaac.2017.03.015

Asarnow, J. R., Goldston, D. B., Tunno, A. M., Inscoe, A. B., & Pynoos, R. (2020). Suicide, self-
harm, & traumatic stress exposure: A trauma-informed approach to the evaluation and management of suicide risk. *Evidence-Based Practice in Child & Adolescent Mental Health*. https://
doi.org/10.1080/23794925.2020.1796547

Coyle, T. N., Shaver, J. A., & Linehan, M. M. (2018). On the potential for iatrogenic effects of
psychiatric crisis services: The example of dialectical behavior therapy for adult women with
borderline personality disorder. *Journal of Consulting and Clinical Psychology, 86*(2), 116.
https://doi.org/10.1037/ccp0000275

Diamond, G. S., Wintersteen, M. B., Brown, G. K., Diamond, G. M., Gallop, R., Shelef, K., & Levy, S. (2010). Attachment-based family therapy for adolescents with suicidal ideation: A randomized controlled trial. *Journal of the American Academy of Child & Adolescent Psychiatry, 49*(2), 122–131. https://doi.org/10.1016/j.jaac.2009.11.002

Esposito-Smythers, C., Spirito, A., Kahler, C. W., Hunt, J., & Monti, P. (2011). Treatment of co-occurring substance abuse and suicidality among adolescents: A randomized trial. *Journal of Consulting and Clinical Psychology, 79*(6), 728. https://doi.org/10.1037/a0026074

Giles, L., Shepard, L., Asarnow, J., & Keeshin, B. R. (2021). Implementation of a trauma -informed suicide prevention intervention for youth presenting to the emergency department in crisis. *Evidence-Based Practice in Child and Adolescent Mental Health, 6*(3), 343–353. https://doi.org/10.1080/23794925.2021.1961643

Glenn, C. R., Esposito, E. C., Porter, A. C., & Robinson, D. J. (2019). Evidence base update of psychosocial treatments for self-injurious thoughts and behaviors in youth. *Journal of Clinical Child & Adolescent Psychology, 48*(3), 357–392. https://doi.org/10.1080/15374416.2019.1591281

Goldston, D. B., & Asarnow, J. R. (2021). Quality improvement for acute trauma-informed suicide prevention care: introduction to special issue. *Evidence-Based Practice in Child and Adolescent Mental Health, 6*, 303–306. https://doi.org/10.1080/23794925.2021.1961645

Hughes, J. L., Anderson, N. L., Wiblin, J. L., & Asarnow, J. R. (2017). Predictors and outcomes of psychiatric hospitalization in youth presenting to the emergency department with suicidality. *Suicide and Life-threatening Behavior, 47*(2), 193–204. https://doi.org/10.1111/sltb.12271

Hutcherson, K., Kennard, B. D., Michaels, M., & Miles, J. (2021). Adapting the safety-acute interventionto improve quality of care for suicidal youth in emergency rooms and medical floors. *Evidence-Based Practice in Child and Adolescent Mental Health, 6*(3), 369–378. https://doi.org/10.1080/23794925.2021.1975516

Jobes, D. A., Vergara, G. A., Lanzillo, E. C., & Ridge-Anderson, A. (2019). The potential use of CAMS for suicidal youth: Building on epidemiology and clinical interventions. *Children's Health Care, 48*(4), 444–468. https://doi.org/10.1080/02739615.2019.1630279

McCauley, E., Berk, M. S., Asarnow, J. R., Adrian, M., Cohen, J., Korslund, K., Avina, C., Hughes, J., Harned, M., Gallop, R., & Linehan, M. M. (2018). Efficacy of dialectical behavior therapy for adolescents at high risk for suicide: A randomized clinical trial. *JAMA Psychiatry, 75*(8), 777–785. https://doi.org/10.1001/jamapsychiatry.2018.1109

Mehlum, L., Ramleth, R. K., Tørmoen, A. J., Haga, E., Diep, L. M., Stanley, B. H., Miller, A. L., Larsson, B., Sund, A. M., & Grøholt, B. (2019). Long term effectiveness of dialectical behavior therapy versus enhanced usual care for adolescents with self-harming and suicidal behavior. *Journal of Child Psychology and Psychiatry, and Allied Disciplines, 60*(10), 1112–1122. https://doi.org/10.1111/jcpp.13077

Ngo, V. K., Asarnow, J. R., Lange, J., Jaycox, L. H., Rea, M. M., Landon, C., Tang, L., & Miranda, J. (2009). Outcomes for youths from racial-ethnic minority groups in a quality improvement intervention for depression treatment. *Psychiatric Services (Washington, DC), 60*(10), 1357–1364. https://doi.org/10.1176/ps.2009.60.10.1357

Perrin, J. M., Asarnow, J. R., Stancin, T., Melek, S. P., & Fritz, G. K. (2019). Mental health conditions and health care payments for children with chronic medical conditions. *Academic Pediatrics, 19*(1), 44–50. https://doi.org/10.1016/j.acap.2018.10.001

Rotheram-Borus, M. J., Piacentini, J., Van Rossem, R., Graae, F., Cantwell, C., Castro-Blanco, D., Miller, S., & Feldman, J. (1996). Enhancing treatment adherence with a specialized emergency room program for adolescent suicide attempters. *Journal of the American Academy of Child and Adolescent Psychiatry, 35*(5), 654–663. https://doi.org/10.1097/00004583-199605000-00021

Rotheram-Borus, M. J., Piacentini, J., Cantwell, C., Belin, T. R., & Song, J. (2000). The 18-month impact of an emergency room intervention for adolescent female suicide attempters. *Journal of Consulting and Clinical Psychology, 68*(6), 1081. https://doi.org/10.1037/0022-006X.68.6.1081

Santamarina-Perez, P., Mendez, I., Singh, M. K., Berk, M., Picado, M., Font, E., Moreno, E., Martínez, E., Morer, A., Borràs, R., Cosi, A., & Romero, S. (2020). Adapted dialectical behavior therapy for adolescents with a high risk of suicide in a community clinic: A pragmatic randomized controlled trial. *Suicide & Life-Threatening Behavior, 50*(3), 652–667. https://doi.org/10.1111/sltb.12612

Stanley, B., Brown, G., Brent, D. A., Wells, K., Poling, K., Curry, J., Kennard, B. D., Wagner, A., Cwik, M. F., Klomek, A. B., Goldstein, T., Vitiello, B., Barnett, S., Daniel, S., & Hughes, J. (2009). Cognitive-behavioral therapy for suicide prevention (CBT-SP): Treatment model, feasibility, and acceptability. *Journal of the American Academy of Child and Adolescent Psychiatry, 48*(10), 1005–1013. https://doi.org/10.1097/CHI.0b013e3181b5dbfe

United States Department of Health and Human Services. (2012). *2012 National Strategy for suicide prevention: Goals and objectives for action*. United States Department of Health and Human Services.

Wu, P., Katic, B. J., Liu, X., Fan, B., & Fuller, C. J. (2010). Mental health service use among suicidal adolescents: Findings from a US national community survey. *Psychiatric Services, 61*(1), 17–24. https://doi.org/10.1176/ps.2010.61.1.17

Zullo, L., Meza, J. I., Rolon-Arroyo, B., Vargas, S., Venables, C., Miranda, J., & Asarnow, J. R. (2020). Enhancing safety: Acute and short-term treatment strategies for youths presenting with suicidality and self-harm. *The Behavior Therapist, 43*(8), 300–304.

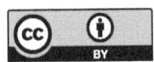

Chapter 9
Safety Planning and Lethal Means Counseling with Youth

Maureen F. Monahan and Barbara Stanley

There is a growing body of research to suggest that most suicidal crises (i.e., the period of time in which someone seriously contemplates killing themselves) are relatively brief. Close to 50% of youth aged 11–15 who died by suicide had no evidence of pre-planning (Holland et al., 2017), and 24% of those aged 13–34 made a near lethal attempt after 5 min of deliberation (Simon et al., 2001). Given that many youth contemplate suicide for a short period of time, targeted interventions during these periods may avert suicide attempts. In particular, having limited access to lethal means and effective methods of distracting from suicidal thoughts and urges play a key role in youth suicide prevention.

One way to thwart suicidal behaviors and allow suicidal crises to dissipate is through the use of a safety plan (SP; Stanley & Brown, 2012; Stanley et al., 2018). SPs are individualized lists of factors that indicate heightened risk of suicide (i.e., warning signs) and ways to prevent the person from engaging in suicidal behaviors. These plans are tailored to individuals at risk and highlight their preferred internal coping strategies, external distractors (i.e., persons and social settings), and contact information for supportive family members, friends, and mental health professionals that can assist during a crisis. Arguably, the most critical component of an SP is lethal means counseling (LMC), the final step in the Stanley-Brown Safety Planning Intervention (Stanley & Brown, 2012), which has been adopted in many healthcare and community settings. LMC involves working directly with individuals at risk for suicide to limit access to lethal methods (e.g., locking pills in a cabinet) until the risk of suicide has diminished substantially. LMC may be especially important for youth living in homes where firearms are present. Studies have documented that youth who live in homes with firearms have up to a fivefold increased risk of

M. F. Monahan (✉) · B. Stanley
New York State Psychiatric Institute, New York, NY, USA

Department of Psychiatry, Columbia University Irving Medical Center, New York, NY, USA
e-mail: Maureen.Monahan@nyspi.columbia.edu; Barbara.Stanley@nyspi.columbia.edu

© The Author(s) 2022
J. P. Ackerman, L. M. Horowitz (eds.), *Youth Suicide Prevention and Intervention*, SpringerBriefs in Psychology,
https://doi.org/10.1007/978-3-031-06127-1_9

suicide, even if they are not the owner of the firearm (for a review see Barber & Miller, 2014). This risk can diminish by 30–50% when firearm access is limited (e.g., temporary removal of firearms from the home, utilizing gun locks), and research suggests limiting access to other lethal means can help further decrease the overall risk of suicide (Barber & Miller, 2014). Thus, LMC in addition to safety planning can have a profound impact on preventing youth suicide.

Safety Planning/Lethal Means Counseling with Youth

An important distinction between youth- and adult-focused suicide-specific treatments (D'Anci et al., 2019) is the emphasis on family involvement, particularly through providing psychoeducation and enhancing family communication and connection. Promising youth treatments that incorporate families include As Safe as Possible (ASAP; Kennard et al., 2018), Cognitive-Behavioral Therapy for Suicide Prevention (CBT-SP; Stanley et al., 2009), the Treatment of Adolescent Suicide Attempters (TASA; Brent et al., 2009), the SAFETY Program (Asarnow et al., 2017), and a specialized emergency room (ER) care intervention (Rotheram-Borus et al., 2000). Family support is a critical component of many successful youth interventions and is also used in the current stand-alone SP interventions for this age group.

Previous work suggests that lethal means interventions that emphasize psychoeducation for parents can significantly increase the likelihood of limiting their child's access to household lethal means (Barber & Miller, 2014). More recent studies have documented positive relationships between SP interventions that involve families and increased outpatient treatment adherence (Asarnow et al., 2011), SP use and means safety behaviors (Hill et al., 2020), and self-efficacy in implementing coping strategies to refrain from suicidal behavior (Czyz et al., 2019). As such, family involvement is likely an important component of youth SP/LMC. Clinical considerations for incorporating families in treatment, as well as other recommendations for engaging in SP/LMC with youth, are discussed below.

Important Considerations for SP/LMC with Youth Clients

Developing an SP with youth clients should always involve a caregiver, either during the development of the plan or after the plan has been created. In either case, caregivers should be provided with copies of their child's SP. This collaboration can increase caregiver self-efficacy in helping youth manage crises and identifying when immediate, emergency care is needed. With caregiver involvement playing a significant role in maintaining safety over time, it is equally as important that youth consent/assent is obtained, and youth are made aware their SP will be shared with their caregivers. Safety planning is built on a foundation of trust between the client and mental health provider. Failing to disclose parent involvement and limitations of confidentiality generally could be perceived as a betrayal of trust with negative implications for treatment adherence and outcomes.

The next set of recommendations relate to the school environment. Similar to working with caregivers, providers should strongly consider communicating with the youth's school regarding their SP and make note of any special accommodations that may be warranted (e.g., unrestricted access to guidance counselors, permission to step out of classroom to use coping skills when highly distressed). Providers should obtain youth consent/assent, make youth clients aware of what will be discussed with the school, and carefully follow each school's unique consenting procedures. Another important consideration is that youth may have different internal coping strategies at school versus at home or outside of school, based on availability of resources and the degree to which each skill can be used covertly (Hill et al., 2020; e.g., deep breathing versus singing aloud versus taking a cold shower). Providers and youth clients may want to develop separate SPs for home and school or create distinct categories for each setting in one comprehensive SP.

It is also important to be aware of how youth's developmental stage may differentially impact the safety planning process. Most youth do not initiate therapy on their own (Stiffman et al., 2004) and may feel a lack of autonomy related to being in treatment in the first place. Without initial buy-in, youth may be less likely to fully engage in therapy, which could negatively impact their likelihood of developing a meaningful SP or disclosing thoughts of suicide. Developmental considerations are especially relevant with respect to counseling on lethal means. SPs should be developed as collaboratively as possible so that the youth feel empowered to have an active role in creating a safe environment rather than restricted. If approached in a prescriptive or rigid manner, clients can interpret a discussion on limiting their access to lethal means as a violation of their rights or a form of punishment. Mental health providers may decide to devote extra time toward reframing this process as a way for the individual to help keep themselves safe, as opposed to a way to restrict their independence.

Fostering the youth's autonomy in this process should be carefully balanced with the overarching goal of keeping them safe. This balance may be more salient when generating lists of internal coping strategies and external supports (Hill et al., 2020). When compared to adults, youth may have less life experience and often a smaller repertoire of coping skills. Thus, providers may have to offer a range of suggestions and teach adaptive coping strategies that will be effective in a time of crisis. In addition, providers should keep in mind the changing peer relationships and perceptions of closeness inherent in adolescence (Marsh et al., 2006). Only adult contacts should be listed as people the youth can turn to for help in a crisis. Trusted peers may only be listed as people who can help *distract* them from suicidal thoughts.

Finally, given the facility youth have with electronic media and its ubiquity, providers should consider utilizing mHealth (mobile health) applications, such as the Stanley-Brown Safety Plan© app (Two Penguins Studios LLC, 2013) or the MY3 app (Mental Health Association of New York City Inc, 2013), in addition to paper copies of the SP. An added benefit of mobile applications is that they are more readily accessible through the youth's phone, as opposed to a paper version which may be more inconvenient or susceptible to being misplaced. It is important to note that these recommendations for youth SP are largely based on clinical judgment and experience as opposed to specific empirical findings. There is a pressing need for research to address the gaps in youth SP.

Future Directions for Research and Policy

Some gaps are methodological and others technological. There is a striking need for studies with rigorous designs (e.g., longitudinal, randomized controlled trials) to assess the effect of youth SP/LMC on key outcomes (e.g., suicidal ideation, attempts, suicides). Along these same lines, future work should investigate the active elements of SP on treatment outcomes to generate a clearer picture of which steps are critical for preventing youth suicide. The field would also benefit from greater development and testing of mHealth or web-based SP interventions for youth. Areas for further study include mobile app push notifications that prompt users to practice coping strategies and reinforcement after successful SP app use to increase the likelihood of using SP strategies in the future. Studying how mobile technologies can increase SP/LMC use is especially relevant in light of the world's growing reliance on technology.

While continued research in these areas is important, SP/LMC practices must also be adopted in real-world settings to effect meaningful change. We are highlighting a call to action to allocate more funding, training, and resources for large-scale implementation and dissemination of SP/LMC across youth educational institutions. Training more school counselors in these brief and effective interventions could have a major impact on youth suicide. Unfortunately, youth at risk often do not get referred for specialized care as suicide risk is complex and sometimes difficult to recognize. Therefore, this initiative would be most effective if, in addition to training school counselors in SP/LMC, training in suicide risk screening was broadly disseminated to school staff and community members (e.g., teachers, administrators, coaches, mentors, etc.). These parallel initiatives could facilitate more referrals to school counselors trained in SP/LMC in the hopes of reducing youth suicide.

Lastly, attention should be paid to care transitions. Youth are at a significantly heightened risk of suicide when transitioning between levels of care (e.g., inpatient unit to outpatient treatment; Fontanella et al., 2020). While SPs can aid in reducing risk during this time, more research and policy work should focus on how healthcare and education systems can work together to make care transitions as safe and seamless as possible.

Conclusion

Research has identified how limiting access to lethal means greatly reduces suicide among adults, yet there is much to learn about SP/LMC with youth clients. Based on what is known regarding current best practices, providers should center SP adaptations around family involvement and strongly consider working with youths' schools to maximize SP efficacy. Providers must also pay careful attention to issues of consent and confidentiality, ensuring that youth are aware of what information will be shared and with whom. Further, providers may decide to devote extra time toward generating buy-in and maintaining a collaborative stance throughout the SP/LMC process. Policy work should focus on care transitions, implementation of SP/LMC in schools, broad dissemination of suicide risk screening in communities, and technological advancement of SP/LMC.

Acknowledgments Research reported in this manuscript was supported by the National Institute of Mental Health of the National Institutes of Health under award numbers R01MH112139 (PI: Stanley) and R01MH109326 (PI: Stanley). The content is solely the responsibility of the authors and does not necessarily represent the official views of the National Institutes of Health.

References

Asarnow, J. R., Baraff, L. J., Berk, M., Grob, C. S., Devich-Navarro, M., Suddath, R., Piancentini, J. C., Rotheram-Borus, M. J., Cohen, D., & Tang, L. (2011). An emergency department intervention for linking pediatric suicidal patients to follow-up mental health treatment. *Psychiatric Services, 62*(11), 1303–1309. https://doi.org/10.1176/ps.62.11.pss6211_1303

Asarnow, J. R., Hughes, J. L., Babeva, K. N., & Sugar, C. A. (2017). Cognitive-behavioral family treatment for suicide attempt prevention: A randomized controlled trial. *Journal of the American Academy of Child & Adolescent Psychiatry, 56*(6), 506–514. https://doi.org/10.1016/j.jaac.2017.03.015

Barber, C. W., & Miller, M. J. (2014). Reducing a suicidal person's access to lethal means of suicide: A research agenda. *American Journal of Preventive Medicine, 47*(3), S264–S272. https://doi.org/10.1016/j.amepre.2014.05.028

Brent, D. A., Greenhill, L. L., Compton, S., Emslie, G., Wells, K., Walkup, J. T., Vitiello, B., Bulstein, O., Stanley, B., Posner, K., Kennard, B., Cwik, M., Wagner, A., Coffery, B., March, J., Riddle, M., Goldstein, T., Curry, J., & Barnett., … Turner, J.B. (2009). The treatment of adolescent suicide attempters study (TASA): Predictors of suicidal events in an open treatment trial. *Journal of the American Academy of Child & Adolescent Psychiatry, 48*(10), 987–996. https://doi.org/10.1097/CHI.0b013e3181b5dbe4

Czyz, E. K., King, C. A., & Biermann, B. J. (2019). Motivational interviewing-enhanced safety planning for adolescents at high suicide risk: A pilot randomized controlled trial. *Journal of Clinical Child & Adolescent Psychology, 48*(2), 250–262. https://doi.org/10.1080/15374416.2018.1496442

D'Anci, K. E., Uhl, S., Giradi, G., & Martin, C. (2019). Treatments for the prevention and management of suicide: A systematic review. *Annals of Internal Medicine, 171*(5), 334–342. https://doi.org/10.7326/M19-0869

Fontanella, C. A., Warner, L. A., Steelesmith, D. L., Brock, G., Bridge, J. A., & Campo, J. V. (2020). Association of timely outpatient mental health services for youths after psychiatric hospitalization with risk of death by suicide. *JAMA Network Open, 3*(8), e2012887. https://doi.org/10.1001/jamanetworkopen.2020.12887

Hill, R. M., Dodd, C. G., Gomez, M., Do, C., & Kaplow, J. B. (2020). The safety planning assistant: Feasibility and acceptability of a web-based suicide safety planning tool for at-risk adolescents and their parents. *Evidence-Based Practice in Child and Adolescent Mental Health, 5*(2), 164–172. https://doi.org/10.1080/23794925.2020.1759469

Holland, K. M., Vivolo-Kantor, A. M., Logan, J. E., & Leemis, R. W. (2017). Antecedents of suicide among youth aged 11–15: A multistate mixed methods analysis. *Journal of Youth and Adolescence, 46*(7), 1598–1610. https://doi.org/10.1007/s10964-016-0610-3

Kennard, B. D., Goldstein, T., Foxwell, A. A., McMakin, D. L., Wolfe, K., Biernesser, C., Morehead, A., Douaihy, A., Zullo, L., Wentroble, E., Owen, V., Zelazny, J., Iyengar, S., Porta, G., & Brent, D. (2018). As Safe as Possible (ASAP): A brief app-supported inpatient intervention to prevent postdischarge suicidal behavior in hospitalized, suicidal adolescents. *American Journal of Psychiatry, 175*(9), 864–872. https://doi.org/10.1176/appi.ajp.2018.17101151

Marsh, P., Allen, J. P., Ho, M., Porter, M., & McFarland, F. C. (2006). The changing nature of adolescent friendships: Longitudinal links with early adolescent ego development. *The Journal of Early Adolescence, 26*(4), 414–431. https://doi.org/10.1177/0272431606291942

Mental Health Association of New York City Inc. (2013). *MY3- Support Network* (Version 5.2) [Mobile application software]. Retrieved from https://apps.apple.com/us/app/my3-support-network/id709651264

Rotheram-Borus, M. J., Piacentini, J., Cantwell, C., Belin, T. R., & Song, J. (2000). The 18-month impact of an emergency room intervention for adolescent female suicide attempters. *Journal of Consulting and Clinical Psychology, 68*(6), 1081. https://doi.org/10.1037//0022-006x.68.6.1081

Simon, T. R., Swann, A. C., Powell, K. E., Potter, L. B., Kresnow, M. J., & O'Carroll, P. W. (2001). Characteristics of impulsive suicide attempts and attempters. *Suicide and Life-threatening Behavior, 32*(Supplement to Issue 1), 49–59. https://doi.org/10.1521/suli.32.1.5.49.24212

Stanley, B., & Brown, G. K. (2012). Safety planning intervention: A brief intervention to mitigate suicide risk. *Cognitive and Behavioral Practice, 19*(2), 256–264. https://doi.org/10.1016/j.cbpra.2011.01.001

Stanley, B., Brown, G., Brent, D., Wells, K., Poling, K., Curry, J., Kennard, B. D., Wagner, A., Cwik, M. F., Klomek, A. B., Goldstein, T., Vitiello, B., Barnett, S., Daniel, S., & Hughes, J. (2009). Cognitive behavior therapy for suicide prevention (CBT-SP): Treatment model, feasibility and acceptability. *Journal of the American Academy of Child and Adolescent Psychiatry, 48*(10), 1005–1013. https://doi.org/10.1097/CHI.0b013e3181b5dbfe

Stanley, B., Brown, G. K., Brenner, L. A., Galfalvy, H. C., Currier, G. W., Knox, K. L., Chaudhury, S. R., Bush, A. L., & Green, K. L. (2018). Comparison of the safety planning intervention with follow-up vs usual care of suicidal patients treated in the emergency department. *JAMA Psychiatry, 75*(9), 894–900. https://doi.org/10.1001/jamapsychiatry.2018.1776

Stiffman, A. R., Pescosolido, B., & Cabassa, L. J. (2004). Building a model to understand youth service access: The gateway provider model. *Mental Health Services Research, 6*(4), 189–198. https://doi.org/10.1023/b:mhsr.0000044745.09952.33

Two Penguins Studios, LLC. (2013). *Stanley-Brown Safety Plan* (Version 2.7) [Mobile application software]. Retrieved from https://apps.apple.com/us/app/stanley-brown-safety-plan/id695122998

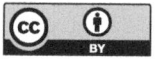

Chapter 10
Youth Crisis Hotlines: Merging Best Practice Suicide Prevention Within a System of Care

Bart Andrews, Laura Coleman, Mandy Bowlin, and Catherine Cox

The primary purpose of a crisis hotline is to provide timely, empathetic support to callers, identify problems and potential solutions, ensure callers are safe, and connect them with appropriate resources. While crisis hotlines can provide support for a variety of presenting concerns, such as domestic abuse or drug use, they are a promising tool for suicide prevention. When individuals experience a suicidal crisis, hotlines can serve as a "just in time" intervention and provide support to ensure immediate safety and a plan for after the crisis resolves.

In 1958, the first suicide prevention crisis hotline in the USA was established in Los Angeles, California (Office of Surgeon General & National Action Alliance, 2012). The line was staffed by trained, community volunteers (Harding, 2009). In 1963, the line began 24/7 coverage, and staff were trained in an active intervention model that emphasized that crises are often short term. Listeners were coached to ask questions such as "Where does it hurt?" and "How can I help?" (Morris, 2011). Subsequently, suicide prevention crisis centers were established throughout the USA to assist those experiencing acute suicidality or emotional distress. In 2004, the Substance Abuse and Mental Health Services Administration (SAMHSA) created the National Suicide Prevention Lifeline (Lifeline), a national network of 180 crisis centers that provides free and confidential emotional support to people in suicidal crisis or emotional distress 24 hours a day, 7 days a week. The Lifeline currently answers over 2 million calls per year (National Suicide Prevention Lifeline, 2020), with call volume likely to increase substantially in the coming years. As of July 16, 2022, "988" is designated as the dialing code for the Lifeline allowing everyone in the USA to quickly access the Lifeline as opposed to the longer 1-800-278-8255 which will remain active as well.

B. Andrews (✉) · L. Coleman · M. Bowlin · C. Cox
Behavioral Health Response (BHR), St. Louis, MO, USA
e-mail: bandrews@bhrworldwide.com; lcoleman@bhrworldwide.com

© The Author(s) 2022
J. P. Ackerman, L. M. Horowitz (eds.), *Youth Suicide Prevention and Intervention*, SpringerBriefs in Psychology,
https://doi.org/10.1007/978-3-031-06127-1_10

Despite the extensive practice of using of crisis hotlines, there are limited data on the prevalence, patterns of use, or overall effectiveness of this type of intervention. Notably, there have been significant challenges in demonstrating the efficacy of crisis hotlines over time, with the most significant being the absence of randomized controlled trials (RCTs) to test effectiveness. However, during the first major expansion of crisis hotlines, a comparison of counties with and without crisis hotlines found evidence that the presence of crisis hotlines was associated with a reduction in suicide rates but only among white women 24 and younger (Miller et al., 1984). Not only is more current effectiveness data needed, but an evaluation of who is willing to access hotlines and who benefits from these interventions is needed.

Crisis hotlines tend to incorporate a similar approach to assisting and managing callers. Generally, an individual experiencing acute distress calls the hotline, and a crisis worker will attempt to de-escalate the situation via phone, create an immediate plan for safety, and, if appropriate, provide referrals to community resources. While this traditional approach has been considered best practice in the field, there are limitations. Prior to the mid-2000s, there was little evidence-based guidance on best practices for suicide prevention and crisis hotline work. For example, "no harm contracts" were considered standard practice at the time despite having no empirical support (Lewis, 2007; see Monahan et al., Chap. 9, this volume).

Although it will be important to augment the research base around crisis hotline interventions over time, we first need to understand the consensus components of best practice in this area. This chapter illustrates innovations in crisis hotline services that can improve the quality of engagement during times when individuals need timely and effective support. Behavioral Health Response (BHR) is a regional crisis hotline located in St. Louis, Missouri. BHR is a member of the National Suicide Lifeline Network and has sought to improve mental health support access for individuals in crisis by adding problem-/demographic-specific hotlines, internet chat links, texting options, telehealth, and mobile outreach responses. This chapter also provides a detailed description of how BHR created and implemented a Youth Connection Helpline system to serve as a model of how to integrate the science of crisis hotline work into a youth-focused community safety net. This chapter emphasizes the importance of integrating crisis hotlines with other community resources and the value of tracking outcomes to achieve intended goals. Guidance on how to implement and evaluate a youth-focused crisis system is provided.

Behavioral Health Response

In 1994, Missouri created a statewide crisis system with 24/7 crisis intervention hotline and mobile outreach services. At the time, Missouri's crisis system was the first statewide crisis system that guaranteed 24/7 telephonic and mobile outreach services that could directly connect callers to state-funded systems of care. Missouri helped to advance the field by using a crisis hotline service to systemically connect callers to both mobile outreach services and ongoing outpatient services. This also marked the beginning of a transition from crisis hotlines being mostly volunteer, community-initiated efforts to publicly funded statewide efforts. As part of this effort, BHR was created to provide crisis hotline and mobile outreach services to residents of the eastern region of Missouri, encompassing St. Louis City and the surrounding nine counties.

BHR provides a regional crisis hotline for the St. Louis metropolitan area and also answers Lifeline calls that originate from this same region. Only about 8% of callers to BHR's regional crisis line report suicidal thoughts compared with the more than 20% of Lifeline callers from the same region. Callers to the regional crisis hotline are often motivated to speak to someone in the moment and establish a connection to services. Alternatively, Lifeline callers are often more motivated to engage in a supportive conversation, are already engaged with services, and often call the Lifeline phone number rather than the crisis line number for their treatment agency. Interestingly, some Lifeline callers struggling with thoughts of suicide avoid calling their own treatment agency's 24/7 crisis line number, as they want to speak to someone outside of their treatment team and want that information kept separate from their ongoing care. It is important to recognize that callers' wants and needs do not always align with providers' wants and needs. Notably, calls to BHR's youth dedicated lines are most often from youth or from a third party (e.g., parent, other concerned adult, peer) trying to obtain help for a youth in crisis.

The BHR Youth Connection Helpline System

The BHR program created the Youth Connection Helpline (YCH) system to better meet the needs of the community. In 2009, only a small percentage of calls, less than 200 callers in all, to BHR were from youth under the age of 18 in a metropolitan area of 2 million people, suggesting limited awareness and/or accessibility. In response, BHR sought and obtained funding to create a youth-focused crisis system in 2010. BHR believed that having a youth-focused line that was dedicated and marketed to youth, with the addition of text and chat access, would increase utilization and lead to more youth in crisis getting services.

In 2010, BHR received a grant from SAMHSA and Lifeline with the aim of adding crisis hotline follow-up services. Prior to receiving this grant, BHR was unable to fund follow-up phone calls. A majority (90%) of crisis calls were resolved via the initial phone call and a referral. The remainder either received a mobile outreach and the case was resolved after completing the mobile outreach. Only callers deemed to require police rescue received follow-up calls and that was to determine outcome of the police response. This grant allowed BHR to make follow-up calls as standard of care for all callers who were experiencing suicide thoughts at the beginning of the call. The results were often dramatic for callers. At first, callers expressed confusion when the option of a follow-up call was offered. However, BHR began reporting deeper and more enriching contact with callers. Because BHR had ongoing contact with an individual after their initial call, BHR was able to better understand how the crisis line had helped them and learn more about the caller's life and their challenges accessing ongoing services. Additionally, BHR clinicians formed more meaningful connections with callers through consistent follow-up. Some client's developed deep bonds with their follow-up clinician, and we had to develop transition plans in order to end the follow-up contact. Offering follow-up phone calls also made it easier to de-escalate callers and decreased use of responses by law enforcement. Callers indicated that the opportunity to receive a follow-up call reduced perceptions of loneliness and created a tangible sense of hope. Collection of outcome data also increased, allowing BHR to track how many callers were connected with mental health services, followed their safety plans, required hospitalization after contact, or subsequently engaged in suicidal behavior.

At the end of 2010, BHR expanded services to all youth under the age of 19 in part of their coverage area, which resulted in the creation of the Youth Connection Helpline (YCH) system. BHR committed to follow up every caller on the YCH, whether the caller was a youth or someone calling about a youth. Additionally, follow-up expanded from 2 weeks (the model of care under the Lifeline follow-up grant) to 4 or 6 weeks. The expansion allowed BHR to add follow-up clinicians whose sole job was to manage outbound follow-up to everyone in follow-up care. Each clinician has a dedicated caseload of follow-up clients so that youth and families speak to the same clinician to maintain continuity. Text and chat options were added over time so that youth could reach the YCH in a mode of their choosing. Mobile outreach services were also expanded so that all callers were eligible for mobile outreach, rather than only the most urgent cases. System of care referrals was built into the electronic health care record so staff could not only see each referral that was provided but, on follow-up, BHR could record each referral that resulted in a service linkage. Outcome variables on every single call are tracked. The YCH thereby became the first fully integrated, 24/7 system of care for youth in the nation.

Best Practices Drive the System

The YCH integrated best practices from Lifeline's standards for assessment and intervention and added non-demand care follow-up for all callers. The standards guiding YCH training include the following: Lifeline Suicide Risk Assessment (Joiner, et al., 2007); Helping Callers at Imminent Risk of Suicide (Draper, et al., 2015); National Suicide Lifeline Follow Up Procedures (National Lifeline, 2021); Counseling on Access to Lethal Means (Frank & Ciocca, 2009); and Stanley and Brown's (2012) Collaborative Suicide Safety Planning.

In addition, all callers received follow-up, including referral sources and any of the caller's active treatment providers. BHR discovered that often the caller's therapist was unaware of the caller's suicide crisis or that when there were multiple providers, the providers were not coordinating care with each other. BHR found that by calling all identified providers and the referral sources, we could improve care coordination and outcomes. YCH follow-up clinicians actively reached out to guardians, teachers, primary care providers, and therapists to ensure clients were linked with appropriate services and everyone in the youth's treatment team was involved with coordinating care. This wraparound approach was key in making sure that it is not just the youth who is the focus of care but that the entire system is responding and adjusting to the needs of the youth. Renaud et al. (2009) found that youth who died of suicide either were not connecting with a care system at all or had inadequate care that was not coordinated across multiple providers and caregivers. The YCH system was designed to ensure callers get established best practices in suicide prevention at each contact using a well-coordinated system-based approach to meet the needs of youth in crisis.

Data and Outcomes

One of the goals of creating the YCH system was to have better data and track the outcomes of our interventions. The following BHR data is from July 1, 2019, to June 30, 2020, and describes the nature of presenting issues, caller responses, and disposition outcomes. Youth-related calls to BHR increased tenfold during the first 3 years of the program. Having youth-specific services (e.g. text, chat, and YCH helpline marketing) significantly increased access to the crisis system. All callers were eligible to participate in the postcrisis follow-up program and 78% (1780/2283) of callers accepted follow-up. A clinical care coordinator contacted callers within 48 hours of their initial call and stayed in touch with the caller on a weekly basis until the crisis was resolved or until the caller decided to no longer participate. The average length of calls between clinical care coordinator and caller was approximately 10 minutes.

The most common presenting problems were non-acute mental health needs such as depression, anxiety, and concentration problems (982/2283), followed by current suicidality (365/2283) and behavioral issues including truancy, running away, risky behaviors, and defiance (320/2283). The most common callers were youth calling for themselves (799/2283); other callers included parents/legal guardians (639/2283), friends/concerned others (502/2283), school staff (159/2283), and social service agency staff (160/2283). Callers reported hearing about YCH from a number of referral sources, including school (753/2283), social service agencies (616/2283), prior use of YCH (410/2283), marketing campaigns (158/2283), family and friends (137/2283), medical providers (114/2283), and police (91/2283).

The majority of calls by YCH were not of immediate life-threatening or acute psychiatric crises, but rather, calls were from youth experiencing significant distress or behavioral disruption with need for in the moment emotional support and connection to services. Providing immediate assistance to parents/guardians, concerned third parties, and agency/school staff also plays an important role in connecting youth to services. School and social service agencies generate the plurality of referrals. Having a system that can support outreach from many different individuals including trusted adults and those who work with youth likely enhances a youth's safety network and ensures that there is no wrong door to getting help.

Of youth accepting follow-up, BHR verified linkage to ongoing care 58% (1032/1780) of the time. These data were especially promising as they also include cases where BHR was unable to reach anyone in follow-up. In cases where BHR did reach someone in follow-up, 72% (1282/1780), linkage to services was verified in 80% (1032/1282) of those cases. Common reasons for failing to connect with ongoing services were that the inability to reach the caller after repeated follow-up attempts (349/498/), declined/discontinued follow-up before linkage verification (125/498), and transportation, insurance, and appointment accessibility issues (25/498).

Several encouraging outcomes emerged; 88% (1566/1780) of clients were diverted from presenting to the emergency department for psychiatric services during follow-up. Of the clients that did present to emergency departments, 75% (160/214) were admitted for inpatient psychiatric treatment. Less than 1% (<18) of clients attempted suicide while receiving follow-up services and there were no reported deaths by suicide.

Case Study: Preteen Suicide

This case study illustrates crisis hotline standards and processes relevant to youth. An elementary school counselor called the YCH after a particularly intense outburst from an 11-year-old girl named Kylie (name and details changed to protect privacy). Kylie recently had several disruptive episodes in class and stated she wanted to kill herself. The phone clinician completed a brief assessment, provided de-escalation support, and recommended a mobile outreach clinician to assist further. The counselor explained they had been unable to reach parents, who were newly divorced and shared custody. A short-term safety plan was developed, and a mobile outreach clinician was dispatched. The phone clinician reached out to both parents and, after a brief dispute, the father agreed to meet the outreach team at the school.

On scene, the clinician completed a detailed risk assessment and determined that the disruptive behaviors had started shortly before the divorce, the distress was serious, but there were no imminent safety concerns or severe symptoms that required inpatient psychiatric care. The clinician developed a collaborative safety plan, ensured the home was free of lethal means of suicide, and referred family for counseling services. The case was transferred to a YCH clinical care coordinator (CCC). The CCC contacted the school and both parents the next day. The school reported that Kylie had not yet scheduled an appointment and the parents provided conflicting accounts of barriers to treatment. After several calls with all three parties, the CCC was able to resolve the communication challenges and arrange a same-day appointment. A week later, Kylie started texting the YCH because she was experiencing thoughts of suicide. The texting clinician reviewed the safety plan with Kylie, connected with her father, ensured immediate safety, and arranged for next-day follow-up. During this follow-up, the CCC contacted all parties, reinforced the safety plan, and made sure the family and treatment agency had a plan in place to address Kylie's needs. After three weekly follow-up calls, the agency was able to confirm ongoing engagement with parents and Kylie with noted improvement. Kylie's parents confirmed she was doing well. No additional texts/calls came through from Kylie. Two weeks later, the CCC followed up with all parties and determined no further assistance was needed.

Recommendations for Youth Connection Helpline Services

In order to establish a feasible and innovative youth connection helpline service, there are several organizational approaches to consider. Continuous quality improvement is key. How youth reach out and the systems that serve youth are ever-changing. It is essential to develop and maintain close relationships with stakeholders, including referring agencies (especially schools) and accepting agencies, law enforcement/juvenile officers, hospitals/urgent care providers, and children and family service organizations. Organizations should also track outcome data such as where callers were referred to, barriers to linkage, use of emergency services, and suicide attempts while in care coordination to improve systems and care. Our experiences with the YCH highlight the importance of follow-up care with callers as well as those who have a role in care coordination. It recommended that care coordinators are available to provide youth with immediate emotional support and resources using a structured approach to follow-up.

Youth connection helpline services should be rooted in a strong evidence base and utilize best practices in service delivery. For instance, it is important to use standardized screening and assessment processes to evaluate suicide risk (see Mournet et al., Chap. 7, this volume) and to minimize coercive interventions whenever possible. Additionally, crisis hotlines for youth should integrate technical strategies to provide alternate modes for crisis contact, such as text, chat, and more structured phone assessment/intervention when mobile outreach services are not available. Using these organizational and technical best practices can allow for the implementation of impactful youth-serving helplines that are able to provide support in times of crisis and allow for connection to potentially lifesaving care.

While suicide prevention via crisis lines has improved, notable gaps still exist. For example, the implementation of 988 has the potential to reshape crisis care across the USA. However, 988 legislation requires states to individually fund 988 services. Without sustained federal support, there are concerns many states may not increase funding to meet 988 and other crisis needs. When the "911" emergency number was rolled out, there was already an existing infrastructure (e.g., law enforcement, jails, ambulances, hospitals) – it was just a matter of making it easier to access those resources. Comparatively, mental healthcare infrastructure is limited and underfunded. If we are going to make significant steps in creating a true system of care, where a call to 988 will lead not only to effective crisis line services but direct and immediate connection to urgent mental health services, national funding will be required to improve the capacity of the crisis systems. Additionally, national funding is needed to create a system of mental health services, from crisis stabilization to urgent mental health clinics and emergency housing. We also need to establish a standard of care that mandates care coordination between providers and verifying linkage to services as opposed to just making a referral. When a clinician makes a referral, it is incumbent upon them to make sure the receiving agency/provider is aware and has accepted the referral. If we do not ensure sustainable, nationwide funding for 988 and enhanced crisis services, we may be creating a highway of crisis line services that dead-end when it is time to connect those callers with ongoing services. A call to a crisis line, in an appropriately funded system, would mean every caller who wanted and needed services would be connected quickly to appropriate ongoing care. Despite progress, we are not there yet.

References

Draper, J., Murphy, G., Vega, E., Covington, D. W., & McKeon, R. (2015). Helping callers to the National Suicide Prevention Lifeline who are at imminent risk of suicide: The importance of active engagement, active rescue, and collaboration between crisis and emergency services. *Suicide & Life-Threatening Behavior, 45*(3), 261–270. https://doi.org/10.1111/sltb.12128

Frank, E. M., & Ciocca, M. (2009). *CALM: Counseling on access to lethal means*. Retrieved May 1, 2020 from https://www.sprc.org/resources-programs/calm-counseling-access-lethal-means-0

Harding, A. (2009). Edwin Schneidman. *The Lancet., 374*, 286. https://doi.org/10.1016/S0140-6736(09)61354-4

Joiner, T., Kalafat, J., Draper, J., Stokes, H., Knudson, M., Berman, A. L., & McKeon, R. (2007). Establishing standards for the assessment of suicide risk among callers to the National Suicide Prevention Lifeline. *Suicide & Life-Threatening Behavior, 37*(3), 353–65. https://doi.org/10.1521/suli.2007.37.3.353

Lewis, L. M. (2007). No-harm contracts: A review of what we know. *Suicide & Life-Threatening Behavior, 37*(1), 50–57. https://doi.org/10.1521/suli.2007.37.1.50

Miller, H. L., Coombs, D. W., Leeper, J. D., & Barton, S. N. (1984). An analysis of the effects of suicide prevention facilities on suicide rates in the United States. *American Journal of Public Health, 74*(4), 340–343. https://doi.org/10.2105/AJPH.74.4.340

Morris, L. (2011) *History of the suicide prevention center, Didi Hirsch Mental Health Services*. Retrieved from http://file.lacounty.gov/SDSInter/dmh/166651_HistoryoftheSuicidePreventionCenter.pdf

National Suicide Prevention Lifeline (2020). *The National Suicide Prevention Lifeline and Alabama*. Retrieved from https://www.sprc.org/sites/default/files/Alabama%20State%20Report%20January-June%202020.pdf

National Suicide Prevention Lifeline (2021) *National Suicide Lifeline Follow Up Guidance* as reference at https://suicidepreventionlifeline.org/wp-content/uploads/2021/05/Follow-Up-Guidance-Doc-2-12.docx.pdf

Office of the Surgeon General (US); National Action Alliance for Suicide Prevention (US). (2012) National Strategy for Suicide Prevention: Goals and Objectives for Action: A Report of the U.S. Surgeon General and of the National Action Alliance for Suicide Prevention. Washington (DC): US Department of Health & Human Services (US); 2012 Sep. Appendix C, Brief History of Suicide Prevention in the United States. Available from: https://www.ncbi.nlm.nih.gov/books/NBK109918/

Renaud, J., Berlim, M. T., Séguin, M., McGirr, A., Tousignant, M., & Turecki, G. (2009). Recent and lifetime utilization of health care services by children and adolescent suicide victims: A case-control study. *Journal of Affective Disorders, 117*(3), 168–173. https://doi.org/10.1016/j.jad.2009.01.004

Stanely, B., & Brown, G. (2012). Safety planning intervention: A brief intervention to mitigate suicide risk. *Cognitive and Behavioral Practice, 19*, 256–264. https://doi.org/10.1016/j.cbpra.2011.01.001

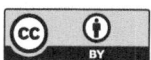

Part IV
Cultural Considerations and Specific Populations

Chapter 11
The Cultural Theory and Model of Suicide for Youth

Joyce Chu, Sam E. O'Neill, Juliana F. Ng, and Oula Khoury

Rates of suicide are often elevated in racial and ethnic minority youth, with increasing rates for Hispanic, Black, and Asian or Pacific Islander youth and a decreasing rate for White youth between 2018 and 2019 (Ramchand et al., 2021). Further, LGBTQ+ youth are at high risk for suicidality, with some research suggesting this population is three times more at risk than their heterosexual and cisgender peers (Hatchel et al., 2021; see Rubin et al., Chap. 13, this volume). These higher suicide rates among racial, ethnic, gender, and sexual minority youth align with some findings that these populations have higher rates of suicide ideation and behaviors, in comparison to their non-minority counterparts (Kann et al., 2016; King et al., 2008). Research has shown that cultural factors play a significant role in predicting and explaining suicidal behavior in racial and ethnic minority youth (Goldston et al., 2008). However, current research has not created recommendations that incorporate cultural considerations for youth, making it difficult for practice and policy to integrate these factors (Polanco-Roman & Miranda, 2021). For this reason, the current chapter presents the Cultural Theory and Model of Suicide for Youth, to provide guidelines for integrating cultural differences into suicide practice, policy, and research.

The Cultural Theory and Model of Suicide for Youth

The original Cultural Theory and Model of Suicide synthesized research from 1991 to 2011 via an extensive literature review of articles regarding culturally specific suicide risk and protective factors into theoretical principles across four major

J. Chu (✉) · S. E. O'Neill · J. F. Ng · O. Khoury
Palo Alto University, Palo Alto, CA, USA
e-mail: jchu@paloaltou.edu; soneill@paloaltou.edu; jng@paloaltou.edu

© The Author(s) 2022
J. P. Ackerman, L. M. Horowitz (eds.), *Youth Suicide Prevention and Intervention*, SpringerBriefs in Psychology,
https://doi.org/10.1007/978-3-031-06127-1_11

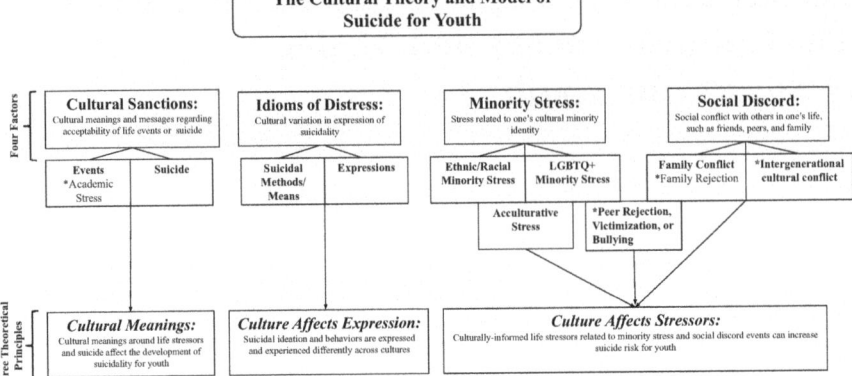

Fig. 11.1 The cultural theory and model of suicide for youth. Author's own creation. (Note: * Indicates additional subdomains added for youth)

cultural factors (cultural sanctions, idioms of distress, minority stress, and social discord). The model was originally developed for use across the life span; however, this chapter examines specific use of the model with cultural minority youth, presented in Fig. 11.1 (Chu et al., 2010). The Cultural Theory and Model of Suicide for Youth addresses the four overarching cultural factors that have been shown in research as particularly salient or more strongly related to suicide behaviors for various ethnic minority and LGBTQ+ youth. Because of this cultural factor rather than group-specific approach, individual minority groups are often discussed together (e.g., as "cultural minority youth") in this chapter.

Cultural Sanctions

Cultural sanctions are the messages of approval or acceptability supported by one's culture. The literature suggests that two types of cultural sanctions, including the unacceptability and shame associated with life events and the acceptability of suicide as an option, influence the developmental pathways to suicide. Notably, cultural sanctions can moderate the relationship between one's exposure to stressful life events and suicidal distress (Chu et al., 2020). For instance, while academic difficulties augment suicide risk for all youth, academic stress is a particularly salient suicide risk factor for Asian American youth due to cultural demands for academic excellence and shame associated with academic failure (Wong et al., 2011).

Second, the perception of suicide as an "acceptable" action increases suicide risk for ethnic and sexual minority youth. For example, some Asian American youth view suicide as a rational (even honorable) way of handling stressful situations that might bring dishonor to their families (Thapa et al., 2015), and lesbian, gay, and bisexual youth have been found to view suicide as more acceptable than their heterosexual counterparts (Canetto et al., 2021). In contrast, religions with negative attitudes toward suicide may protect ethnic minority youth from suicide risk (Cole-Lewis et al., 2016).

Idioms of Distress

A second major way in which culture interfaces with suicide risk is through variations in youth's expression of suicidal distress – called "idioms of suicidal distress." Chu et al. (2010) suggested that minoritized individuals vary in whether or not they express suicidal thoughts and behaviors, the manner of expression, and specific methods of attempting suicide. Ethnic minority youth, for example, appear to be less likely to reveal their suicidal ideation and behaviors (Anderson et al., 2015). Externalizing behaviors as an effort to guard themselves against victimization may be particularly related to suicide expression among Black youth (Congressional Black Caucus Emergency Taskforce on Black Youth Suicide and Mental Health, 2019). As another example, Latinx youth tend to express their suicidality through risk-taking behaviors, irritability, and substance use (Olshen et al., 2007).

Minority Stress

Minority stress includes elevated stress levels stemming from experiences of discrimination and social inequities for youth of minority status (Meyer, 2003). Such stress results in increased depression, substance use, and suicidal thoughts or behaviors. For Black youth, discrimination, racism, low socioeconomic status, and neighborhood disadvantage are associated with higher risk of suicidal thoughts and behaviors (Opara et al., 2020). Among Asian American youth, experiences of perceived discrimination have been linked to increased lifetime suicidal ideation and attempts (Kuroki & Tilley, 2012). Likewise, experiences of victimization and prejudice among transgender individuals (particularly for ages below 25) are related to high levels of suicidality (Johns et al., 2019). Research has also shown that acculturative stress from both family and society is positively associated with suicidal thoughts and behaviors in Latinx, Asian American, and Black youth (Gomez et al., 2011).

Social Discord

Family discord, conflict, perceived burdensomeness, and lack of positive relationships are strong predictors of suicide risk for Hispanic, Asian American, and Black youth (Garza & Pettit, 2010; Joe et al., 2007; Kuroki & Tilley, 2012). Intergenerational cultural conflict (ICC) is a unique construct associated with family discord, which refers to the gaps between levels of acculturation and cultural values between youth and their parents. This conflict is shown to be a stronger contributing factor to Latinx and Asian American youth's suicide behaviors in comparison to their White counterparts (Fortuna et al., 2007; Lau et al., 2002). Additionally, family alienation and invalidating familial discourse are related to increased suicidal thoughts and behaviors for LGBTQ+ youth (McBee-Strayer & Rogers, 2002).

Peer rejection, victimization, and bullying are also strongly associated with an increased risk of suicidal behaviors among LGBTQ+ youth with ethnic minority identities (Hatchel et al., 2019a, b). The relationship between peer victimization/bullying and suicidal ideation is mediated by increased feelings of alienation and a reduced sense of school belonging (Lardier et al., 2020).

Three Theoretical Principles for Cultural Suicide Factors

Past research indicates that the four cultural suicide factors - cultural sanctions, idioms of distress, minority stress, and social discord - operate according to the following three theoretical principles. First, culture affects the types of stressors that are related to increased suicidal ideation and behaviors for youth. Second, the cultural meanings (i.e., cultural sanctions) associated with life stressors and suicide affect the development of suicide risk, one's threshold of tolerance for psychological pain, and potential for suicidal behavior. Third, culture affects how suicidal thoughts and behaviors are expressed. In particular, culture can impact how one expresses their suicidality, such as their choice to disclose or hide their thoughts, as well as what methods they use to make attempts.

Implications

Practice Implications

Given the myriad of ways that suicidal distress can be expressed across cultures, cultural idioms of suicidal distress should be integrated into screening and assessment for symptoms of suicidal ideation, intent, plan, and means. For example, the Cultural Assessment of Risk for Suicide (CARS; Chu et al., 2013) was developed to assess culturally specific suicide risk factors among adults, which is now adapted, but not yet psychometrically validated, for use with adolescents as CARS-A (Khoury, 2020). Furthermore, how youth symptoms are assessed (e.g., interview and self-report), what questions are asked and in what sequence, and how confidentiality concerns and psychoeducation are provided should be carefully considered. Providers need to account for internalized stigma, trust with healthcare systems, different reporting styles, willingness to disclose risk, and unique idioms or expressions of suicidal distress for ethnic, gender, and sexual minority youth. Moreover, risk and protective factors related to minority stress and social discord should be integrated into comprehensive assessment protocols to determine the ultimate suicide risk level for clients, with cultural sanctions/meanings of suicide about stressors and suicide as influential factors that modulate such risk. Together, these factors and principles are important for facilitating recovery through culturally tailored safety plans and treatments with youth and their families.

Research Implications

The four factors and three principles of the Cultural Theory and Model of Suicide for Youth can serve as grounding principles for research across diverse populations. It is important to use evidence-based tools and assessments to ensure consistency across the field and that all individuals are screened appropriately. Studies are needed to further develop and validate culturally adapted suicide risk screening and assessment measures for adolescents, as well as to infuse these cultural factors into adaptations of existing evidence-based protocols. There is also a growing need to validate, adapt, or create suicide prevention programs that are specifically tailored to these factors. Future research is needed to deepen our understanding of the ways in which the cultural factors and principles are experienced in specific cultural groups. This research has particular relevance for cultural minority subgroups who have elevated rates and/or risk for suicide, suicidal ideation, or attempts (e.g., Latinx, Black, Native American/Alaskan Native, and LGBTQ+ youth).

Policy Implications

Suicide prevention strategic plans and safety protocols at the school, county, state, and national level should incorporate culture and diversity (including the four factors and three principles of the Cultural Theory and Model of Suicide for Youth identified in this chapter) as a priority when aiming to reduce youth suicide. For example, policies outlining best practices for suicide prevention efforts should include targeted outreach to specific groups of minoritized youth experiencing family rejection and/or academic stress. Prevention and postvention services in schools should also incorporate minority-specific resources (e.g., The Trevor Project for LGBTQ+ youth). Furthermore, resources that include suicide warning signs should highlight cultural factors (e.g., idioms of distress such as risk-taking behaviors, irritability, or displays of aggression, or minority stress such as feeling targeted or bullied as a minority individual) to promote awareness of specific cues for minority youth suicide risk.

Training and education policies would also benefit from integration with the Cultural Theory and Model of Suicide for Youth. For example, policymakers and administrators should place a strong value on cultural factors as they prioritize suicide-related competencies in mental health graduate education, and state-level licensing requirements that require continuing education in suicide. Otherwise, well-meaning efforts may fall short of meeting the needs of some of our most vulnerable youth and families. Finally, local and national guidelines for suicide safety and treatment should be re-examined from a cultural lens taking into account the factors highlighted throughout this chapter and a willingness to revise or recreate programs.

Conclusions

Evidence, although limited, suggests that a downward extension of the Cultural Theory and Model of Suicide is appropriate for ethnic, gender, and sexual minority youth, with considerations of specific risk factors that may increase their vulnerability to suicidal behaviors. A better understanding about how risk factors such as academic stress, ICC, and peer rejection influence suicide risk can have implications for practice, research, and policy. Routine integration of these cultural risk and protective factors of suicide will help promote cultural responsivity in youth suicide prevention and postvention efforts. Recent efforts to attend to the need for cultural infusion into suicide prevention efforts are evident in printed resources such as the Suicide Prevention Resource Center's Guidelines for Culturally and Linguistically Responsive Media & Resource Materials or Guidance for Culturally Adapting Gatekeeper Trainings (SPRC, 2017, 2020); however, progress is nascent and in need of dedicated commitment and resources in the field. There is an urgent need to provide additional support for practitioners, researchers, and policymakers to further integrate culture into the valuable work of mitigating youth suicidality.

References

Anderson, L. M., Lowry, L. S., & Wuensch, K. L. (2015). Racial differences in adolescents' answering questions about suicide. *Death Studies, 39*(10), 600–604. https://doi.org/10.108 0/07481187.2015.1047058

Canetto, S. S., Antonelli, P., Ciccotti, A., Dettore, D., & Lamis, D. A. (2021). Suicidal as normal – A lesbian, gay, and bisexual youth script? *Crisis, 42*(4), 292–300. https://doi.org/10.1027/0227-5910/a000730

Chu, J. P., Goldblum, P., Floyd, R., & Bongar, B. (2010). The cultural theory and model of suicide. *Applied and Preventive Psychology, 14*, 25–40. https://doi.org/10.1016/j.appsy.2011.11.001

Chu, J., Floyd, R., Diep, H., Pardo, S., Goldblum, P., & Bongar, B. (2013). A tool for the culturally competent assessment of suicide: The Cultural Assessment of Risk for Suicide (CARS) measure. *Psychological Assessment, 25*(2), 424–434. https://doi.org/10.1037/a0031264

Chu, J., Maruyama, B., Batchelder, H., Goldblum, P., Bongar, B., & Wickham, R. E. (2020). Cultural pathways for suicidal ideation and behaviors. *Cultural Diversity & Ethnic Minority Psychology, 26*(3), 367–377. https://doi.org/10.1037/cdp0000307

Cole-Lewis, Y. C., Gipson, P. Y., Opperman, K. J., Arango, A., & King, C. A. (2016). Protective role of religious involvement against depression and suicidal ideation among youth with interpersonal problems. *Journal of Religion and Health, 55*(4), 1172–1188. https://doi.org/10.1007/s10943-016-0194-y

Fortuna, L. R., Perez, D. J., Canino, G., Sribney, W., & Alegria, M. (2007). Prevalence and correlates of lifetime suicidal ideation and suicide attempts among Latino subgroups in the United States. *The Journal of Clinical Psychiatry, 68*(4), 572–581. https://doi.org/10.4088/jcp.v68n0413

Garza, M. J., & Pettit, J. W. (2010). Perceived burdensomeness, familism, and suicidal ideation among Mexican women: Enhancing understanding of risk and protective factors. *Suicide & Life-Threatening Behavior, 40*(6), 561–573. https://doi.org/10.1521/suli.2010.40.6.561

Goldston, D. B., Molock, S. D., Whitbeck, L. B., Murakami, J. L., Zayas, L. H., & Nagayama Hall, G. C. (2008). Cultural considerations in adolescent suicide prevention and psychosocial treatment. *The American Psychologist, 63*(1), 14–31. https://doi.org/10.1037/0003-066X.63.1.14

Gomez, J., Miranda, R., & Polanco, L. (2011). Acculturative stress, perceived discrimination, and vulnerability to suicide attempts among emerging adults. *Journal of Youth and Adolescence, 40*(11), 1465–1476. https://doi.org/10.1007/s10964-011-9688-9

Hatchel, T., Delgado, A. V., Huang, Y., & Espelage, D. L. (2019a). Minority stress among transgender adolescents: The role of peer victimization, school belonging, and ethnicity. *Journal of Child and Family Studies, 28*, 2467–2476. https://doi.org/10.1007/s10826-018-1168-3

Hatchel, T., Ingram, K. M., Mintz, S., Hartley, C., Valido, A., Espelage, D. L., & Wayman, P. (2019b). Predictors of suicidal ideation and attempts among LGBTQ adolescents: The roles of help-seeking beliefs, peer victimization, depressive symptoms, and drug use. *Journal of Child and Family Studies, 28*, 2443–2455. https://doi.org/10.1007/s10826-019-01339-2

Hatchel, T., Polanin, J. R., & Espelage, D. L. (2021). Suicidal thoughts and behaviors among LGBTQ youth: Meta-analyses and a systematic review. *Archives of Suicide Research, 25*(1), 1–37. https://doi.org/10.1080/13811118.2019.1663329

Joe, S., Romer, D., & Jamieson, P. E. (2007). Suicide acceptability is related to suicide planning in U.S. adolescents and young adults. *Suicide and Life-threatening Behavior, 37*(2), 165–178. https://doi.org/10.1521/suli.2007.37.2.165

Johns, M. M., Lowry, R., Andrzejewski, J., Barrios, L. C., Demissie, Z., McManus, T., Rasberry, C. N., Robin, L., & Underwood, J. M. (2019). Transgender identity and experiences of violence victimization, substance use, suicide risk, and sexual risk behaviors among high school students—19 states and large Urban School districts, 2017. *Morbidity and Mortality Weekly Report, 68*(3), 67–71. https://doi.org/10.15585/mmwr.mm6803a3

Kann, L., McManus, T., Harris, W. A., Shanklin, S. L., Flint, K. H., Hawkins, J., et al. (2016). Youth risk behavior surveillance—United States, 2015. *Morbidity and Mortality Weekly Report. Surveillance Summaries (Washington, DC: 2002), 65*(6), 1–174.

Khoury, O. (2020). Adaptation of the cultural assessment of risk for suicide measure for adolescents [ProQuest Information & Learning]. In Dissertation abstracts international: Section B: The sciences and engineering, vol. 81, issue 2–B

King, M., Semlyen, J., Tai, S. S., Killaspy, H., Osborn, D., Popelyuk, D., & Nazareth, I. (2008). A systematic review of mental disorder, suicide, and deliberate self harm in lesbian, gay and bisexual people. *BMC Psychiatry, 8*, 70. https://doi.org/10.1186/1471-244X-8-70

Kuroki, Y., & Tilley, J. L. (2012). Recursive partitioning analysis of lifetime suicidal behaviors in Asian Americans. *Asian American Journal of Psychology, 3*(1), 17–28. https://doi.org/10.1037/a0026586

Ladier, D. T., Pinto, S. A., Brammer, M. K., Garcia-Reid, P., & Reid, R. J. (2020). The relationship between queer identity, social connection, school bullying, and suicidal ideations among youth of color. *Journal of LGBT Issues in Counseling, 14*, 74–99.

Lau, A. S., Jernewall, N. M., Zane, N., & Myers, H. F. (2002). Correlates of suicidal behaviors among Asian American outpatient youths. *Cultural Diversity & Ethnic Minority Psychology, 8*(3), 199–213. https://doi.org/10.1037/1099-9809.8.3.199

McBee-Strayer, S. M., & Rogers, J. R. (2002). Lesbian, gay, and bisexual suicidal behavior: Testing a constructivist model. *Suicide & Life-Threatening Behavior, 32*(3), 272–283. https://doi.org/10.1521/suli.32.3.272.22171

Meyer, I. H. (2003). Prejudice, social stress, and mental health in lesbian, gay, and bisexual populations: Conceptual issues and research evidence. *Psychological Bulletin, 129*(5), 674–697. https://doi.org/10.1037/0033-2909.129.5.674

Olshen, E., McVeigh, K. H., Wunsch-Hitzig, R. A., & Rickert, V. I. (2007). Dating violence, sexual assault, and suicide attempts among urban teenagers. *Archives of Pediatrics & Adolescent Medicine, 161*(6), 539. https://doi.org/10.1001/archpedi.161.6.539

Opara, I., Assan, M. A., Pierre, K., Gunn, J. F., Metzger, I., Hamilton, J., & Arugu, E. (2020). Suicide among Black children: An integrated model of the interpersonal-psychological theory of suicide and intersectionality theory for researchers and clinicians. *Journal of Black Studies, 51*(6), 611–631. https://doi.org/10.1177/0021934720935641

Polanco-Roman, L., & Miranda, R. (2021). A cycle of exclusion that impedes suicide research among racial and ethnic minority youth. *Suicide and Life-threatening Behavior, 52,* 171–174. https://doi.org/10.1111/sltb.12752

Ramchand, R., Gordon, J. A., & Pearson, J. L. (2021). Trends in suicide rates by race and ethnicity in the United States. *JAMA Network Open, 4*(5). https://doi.org/10.1001/jamanetworkopen.2021.11563

Suicide Prevention Resource Center. (2017). *Creating linguistically and culturally competent suicide prevention materials.* Education Development Center, Inc.

Suicide Prevention Resource Center. (2020). *Guidance for culturally adapting gatekeeper trainings.* Education Development Center, Inc.

Thapa, P., Sung, Y., Klingbeil, D. A., Lee, C. Y., & Klimes-Dougan, B. (2015). Attitudes and perceptions of suicide and suicide prevention messages for Asian Americans. *Behavioral Sciences (Basel, Switzerland), 5*(4), 547–564. https://doi.org/10.3390/bs5040547

The Congressional Black Caucus (CBC), Emergency Taskforce on Black Youth Suicide and Mental Health. (2019). *Ring the alarm: The crisis of black youth suicide in America.* https://watsoncoleman.house.gov/uploadedfiles/full_taskforce_report.pdf

Wong, Y. J., Brownson, C., & Schwing, A. E. (2011). Risk and protective factors associated with Asian American students' suicidal ideation: A multicampus, national study. *Journal of College Student Development, 52*(4), 396–408.

Chapter 12
Black Youth Suicidal Behavior: What We Know and Where We Go from Here

Arielle H. Sheftall and Rhonda C. Boyd

There is a crisis among Black youth that has largely been ignored. A racial disparity in youth suicide and suicidal behavior (SIB) has been found (Bridge et al., 2015; Lindsey et al., 2019; Sheftall et al., 2016), yet little research, policy, or practice recommendations have been suggested to address these gaps. This limits our ability to prevent the devastating effects of suicide and SIB in Black communities.

The limited data we do have suggest Black children experience elevated suicide risk compared to the general population. Specifically, Bridge et al. (2015) identified a significant increase for suicide rates for Black males, while a decrease was seen in their White counterparts over the course of two decades from 1993 to 2012. A follow-up study examined precipitating circumstances of suicide found child (5–11 years) decedents were more likely to be Black compared to early adolescent (12–14 years) decedents (Sheftall et al., 2016). Finally, in a recent publication investigating SIB in high school youth, researchers found from 1991 to 2017 suicide attempts increased 73% in Black adolescents and, for Black males, an increase of 122% was found for suicide attempts requiring medical care, suggesting a higher lethality for suicide attempts for this group of youth (Lindsey et al., 2019).

The increase in SIB among Black youth is disturbing, and the reasons behind these increases are unclear and in need of further investigation. In 2019, the

A. H. Sheftall (✉)
The Center for Suicide Prevention and Research at the Abigail Wexner Research Institute at Nationwide Children's Hospital, Department of Pediatrics at the Ohio State University Medical Center, Columbus, OH, USA
e-mail: Arielle.Sheftall@nationwidechildrens.org

R. C. Boyd
Department of Child and Adolescent Psychiatry and Behavioral Sciences at the Children's Hospital of Philadelphia and the University of Pennsylvania Perelman School of Medicine, Philadelphia, PA, USA
e-mail: rboyd@pennmedicine.upenn.edu

© The Author(s) 2022
J. P. Ackerman, L. M. Horowitz (eds.), *Youth Suicide Prevention and Intervention*, SpringerBriefs in Psychology,
https://doi.org/10.1007/978-3-031-06127-1_12

Congressional Black Caucus convened an Emergency Taskforce on Black Youth Suicide and Mental Health, and its workgroup of researchers, clinicians, and public health officials issued the "Ring the Alarm" report which described the problem of Black youth suicide and set forth recommendations for research, practice, and policy (Congressional Black Caucus Emergency Taskforce on Black Youth Suicide and Mental Health, 2019). The current article extends this seminal report's recommendations and provides additional perspectives relevant to addressing the current crisis of Black youth SIB.

Research Recommendations

There is a dearth of research studies that focus on Black youth SIB and prevention strategies. Research studies should not assume that prior work done with primarily White middle-class youth will generalize, but rather they may need to start from the ground level and work toward suicide prevention strategies specific to Black youth (Sheftall & Miller, 2021). We must first understand the risk (e.g., racial discrimination (Opara et al., 2020)) and protective factors (e.g., high faith-based community involvement (Molock et al., 2008)) that are specific for Black youth. This understanding will have repercussions on the specific suicide prevention strategies used.

A major challenge is that the current lens we use for suicide prevention may be inappropriate for Black youth (Bath & Njoroge, 2021). Suicide prevention methods that incorporate principles of justice, equity, diversity, and inclusion (JEDI; Bath & Njoroge, 2021) will lead to more culturally sensitive prevention methods. JEDI offers a perspective of being conscious about race/ethnicity and racism that Black youth encounter regularly. The lack of their incorporation within suicide prevention research undermines the experiences of Black youth and limits our ability to advance the field. However, implementation and testing of programs that incorporate these principles through randomized controlled trials (RCTs) has not been conducted. Doing so would provide improved understanding of what works for preventing SIB in Black youth.

Another recommendation for research is to test how engaging community members and other institutions in the prevention of SIB could be beneficial in decreasing the rates among Black youth. For example, prevention strategies for medical concerns (e.g., hypertension) for Black men have been implemented in places outside of healthcare settings such as barbershops (Ferdinand et al., 2020) and have been highly successful. However, for youth SIB the literature is limited. One study suggests there is value in incorporating the church into youth suicide prevention (Molock et al., 2008); however, large-scale studies are still needed to determine if this is an avenue Black youth suicide prevention should take. Finally, examining the effectiveness of existing evidence-based suicide prevention programs with Black youth populations, then adapting these suicide preventive interventions to meet the specific needs of Black youth, and testing these adaptations are research gaps that must be filled.

Practice Recommendations

The increased risk for SIBs for Black children and adolescents signals an urgent need for action. Despite the limited research, Black youth must be provided services to treat SIBs and prevent deaths. There are multiple settings (e.g., primary care, emergency departments, schools, juvenile justice, child welfare) in which youth are identified to be at increased risk for suicide and provided services. Suicide prevention efforts should be implemented in all of them to varying degrees. Three practice-related areas to be discussed in the context of Black youth suicide include (1) identification, (2) mental health utilization disparities, and (3) intervention.

Identification

One critical issue is the accurate identification of suicide risk in Black youth. Although there are not screening questions developed specifically for Black youth, it is important to routinely ask Black youth about SIB. Recent findings suggest for Black youth, parents are more likely to be unaware of youth's suicidal ideation and youth are more likely to deny suicidal ideation that parents report (Jones et al., 2019). We need to improve understanding of Black youth reporting patterns. This raises concern that providers may be missing SIB risk (DeVylder et al., 2019), especially if they rely solely on parent report or lack knowledge of current trends, risks, and behavioral presentations for Black youth.

Additionally, providers should consider risk, protective, and cultural factors that impact youth's potential for SIBs (Opara et al., 2020). It is critical that providers are aware that exposure to racism and discrimination, community violence exposure, and trauma occur disproportionately among Black youth and can serve as risk factors for SIBs (Congressional Black Caucus Emergency Taskforce on Black Youth Suicide and Mental Health, 2019). Thus, inquiring about such factors in clinical assessments is necessary (Opara et al., 2020). Inquiring about protective factors such as religious affiliation, extended family support, and community assets among others is significant to complete clinical formulation and to be incorporated into safety planning. Gathering this clinical information for Black youth and their families should inform treatment, the planning of services, and cannot be overlooked.

Mental Health Utilization Disparities

There is a longstanding disparity in mental health service utilization among Black youth (Freedenthal, 2007). Two recent systematic reviews examined why this lack of utilization may exist (Fante-Coleman & Jackson-Best, 2020; Planey et al., 2019). The most relevant factors included lack of perceived need, self-reliance, mental health stigma, mistrust of providers and treatment, perception of treatment effectiveness, few mental health centers present, difficulties in physically accessing available services (e.g., transportation), and associated costs and insurance limitations. Furthermore, clinician barriers included a lack of cultural competence and bias (Fante-Coleman & Jackson-Best, 2020; Planey et al., 2019). These reviews also identified factors that could facilitate mental health service engagement for Black youth. Preliminary findings suggest that severity of mental health presentation, supportive social network, parental expectations and experiences, and referrals from those the family/youth feel comfortable with may increase engagement (Fante-Coleman & Jackson-Best, 2020; Planey et al., 2019). It is crucial for providers and practices to address these barriers strategically to improve engagement in mental health services for Black youth.

Intervention

Currently, providers are tasked with treating Black youth for suicide risk using limited empirical evidence. Promising treatments for suicidal outcomes with Black youth include multisystemic therapy and attachment-based family therapy. However, large-scale trials with Black youth have not been implemented to date (Congressional Black Caucus Emergency Taskforce on Black Youth Suicide and Mental Health, 2019). Robinson et al. (2016) culturally adapted an empirically based cognitive behavioral depression prevention for Black adolescents with suicide risk in a school setting. The intervention was associated with a reduction in suicide risk compared to standard care. Additionally, there is a need to identify alternative settings and ways to deliver services for Black youth. Providing services in community settings with partnerships with the community stakeholders should be explored. These community mental health services must be easily accessible and trustworthy for Black youth. Also, mental health check-in slots can be available in these settings so youth who are experiencing an acute stressor can receive immediate assistance and triage as an alternative to an emergency department setting prior to SIBs.

When providing mental health services for Black youth, culturally competent mental health care without bias and racism is critical. Doing this effectively involves training providers to be culturally competent in assessment and treatment of Black youth. Moreover, providers need to incorporate culturally specific risk and protective factors into the delivery of interventions and programs (Opara et al., 2020). Graduate training programs, professional societies, and licensing organizations can be utilized to provide in-depth trainings in these domains. Furthermore, we recommend that it is required for professional license renewal to participate in training focused on cultural competence with Black individuals. For practices, it is critical to identify Black youth suicide prevention as a priority. Directors of practices should ensure quality improvement projects are conducted to directly measure how responsive providers' services are for Black youth with suicide risk. To support this, funding for practice-based and quality improvement projects is needed as well as supports to dissemination.

Policy Recommendations

Current policies have not addressed Black youth suicide or mental health disparities. We will not make advances in mental health and suicide outcomes for Black youth without having intentional policies targeting this problem. On a positive note, a few activities have recently been initiated to address Black youth suicide. The Pursuing Equity in Mental Health Act (H.R. 1475; Watson Coleman, 2021) was introduced into Congress. The bill seeks to advance integrated behavioral health programs, increase mental health disparity research, establish professional competencies to address racial/ethnic disparities, and develop a behavioral health outreach and education program. Also, the Mental Health Services for Students Act of 2020 (H.R. 1109; Napolitano, 2019) seeks to amend the current Public Health Service Act to increase access to and availability of comprehensive mental health interventions in school settings. To complement these acts, we recommend further investments into Black communities and partnerships with community organizations to focus specifically on Black youth and to provide more culturally competent mental health services for Black youth with suicide risk.

Conclusion

Black clinicians and academics are underrepresented to advance this work. For example, only 4% of psychologists in the workforce are Black, although increases are present for early career psychologists (11%; Lin et al., 2018). Additionally, Black researchers are less likely to receive large grant funding (e.g., R01) from the National Institutes of Health compared to their White counterparts (Hoppe et al., 2019). To combat these problems, we recommend formulating a Black Youth Mental Health and SIB Consortium. This consortium would include a multidisciplinary group of experts that would confront the problem of Black youth suicide and would be available to provide training and expertise across research, practice, and policy settings. A funded consortium would address the above recommendations for the discovery of effective methods to engage Black individuals into the behavioral health workforce, advance our knowledge concerning Black youth mental health and SIB, and provide guidance concerning policies geared toward Black youth mental health.

Acknowledgments We would like to thank all the members of the Congressional Black Caucus Emergency Taskforce on Black Youth Suicide and Mental Health and its workgroup that worked together under the leadership of Representative Bonnie Watson Coleman to write a comprehensive report concerning Black youth suicide and mental health.

Funding Details Dr. Sheftall is supported by the National Institute of Mental Health (NIMH; R21MG116206) and the American Foundation for Suicide Prevention (AFSP; YIG-1-152-19). Dr. Boyd is supported by the National Institute of Mental Health (P50MH127511) and the Deneen and Coyle Suicide Prevention Center Fund. None of the funders were involved in manuscript preparation.

References

Bath, E., & Njoroge, W. F. M. (2021). Coloring outside the lines: Making black and brown lives matter in the prevention of youth suicide. *Journal of the American Academy of Child and Adolescent Psychiatry, 60*(1), 17–21. https://doi.org/10.1016/j.jaac.2020.09.013

Bridge, J. A., Asti, L., Horowitz, L. M., Greenhouse, J. B., Fontanella, C. A., Sheftall, A. H., Kelleher, K. J., & Campo, J. V. (2015). Suicide trends among elementary school-aged children in the United States from 1993 to 2012. *JAMA Pediatrics, 169*(7), 673–677. https://doi.org/10.1001/jamapediatrics.2015.0465

Congressional Black Caucus Emergency Taskforce on Black Youth Suicide and Mental Health. (2019). *Ring the alarm: The crisis of black youth suicide in America.* Retrieved from https://watsoncoleman.house.gov/uploadedfiles/full_taskforce_report.pdf

DeVylder, J. E., Ryan, T. C., Cwik, M., Wilson, M. E., Jay, S., Nestadt, P. S., Goldstein, M., & Wilcox, H. C. (2019). Assessment of selective and universal screening for suicide risk in a pediatric emergency department. *JAMA Network Open, 2*(10), e1914070–e1914070. https://doi.org/10.1001/jamanetworkopen.2019.14070

Fante-Coleman, T., & Jackson-Best, F. (2020). Barriers and facilitators to accessing mental healthcare in Canada for black youth: A scoping review. *Adolescent Research Review, 5*, 115–136. https://doi.org/10.1007/s40894-020-00133-2

Ferdinand, D. P., Nedunchezhian, S., & Ferdinand, K. C. (2020). Hypertension in African Americans: Advances in community outreach and public health approaches. *Progress in Cardiovascular Diseases, 63*(1), 40–45. https://doi.org/10.1016/j.pcad.2019.12.005

Freedenthal, S. (2007). Racial disparities in mental health service use by adolescents who thought about or attempted suicide. *Suicide & Life-Threatening Behavior, 37*(1), 22–34. https://doi.org/10.1521/suli.2007.37.1.22

Hoppe, T., Litovitz, A., Willis, K., Meseroll, R., Perkins, M., Hutchins, B., Davis, A., Lauer, M., Valantine, H., Anderson, J., & Santangelo, G. (2019). Topic choice contributes to the lower rate of NIH awards to African-American/black scientists. *Science Advances, 5*(10), 7238. https://doi.org/10.1126/sciadv.aaw7238

Jones, J. D., Boyd, R. C., Calkins, M. E., Ahmed, A., Moore, T. M., Barzilay, R., Benton, T. D., & Gur, R. E. (2019). Parent adolescent agreement about adolescents' suicidal thoughts. *Pediatrics, 143*(2). https://doi.org/10.1542/peds.2018-1771

Lin, L., Stamm, K., & Christidis, P. (2018). How diverse is the psychology workforce? *Monitor on Psychology, 49*(2), 19.

Lindsey, M., Sheftall, A., Xiao, Y. Y., & Joe, S. (2019). Trends of suicidal behaviors among high school students in the United States: 1991-2017. *Pediatrics, 144*(5). https://doi.org/10.1542/peds.2019-1187

Molock, S. D., Matlin, S., Barksdale, C., Puri, R., & Lyles, J. (2008). Developing suicide prevention programs for African American youth in African American churches. *Suicide & Life-Threatening Behavior, 38*(3), 323–333. https://doi.org/10.1521/suli.2008.38.3.323

Napolitano, G. F. (2019). *H.R.1109-Mental health services for students act 2020.* https://www.congress.gov/bill/116th-congress/house-bill/1109?q=%7B%22search%22%3A%5B%22mental+health%22%5D%7D&r=3&s=1

Opara, I., Assan, M. A., Pierre, K., Gunn, J. F., Metzger, I., Hamilton, J., & Arugu, E. (2020). Suicide among black children: An integrated model of the interpersonal-psychological theory of suicide and intersectionality theory for researchers and clinicians. *Journal of Black Studies, 51*(6), 611–631. https://doi.org/10.1177/0021934720935641

Planey, A. M., Smith, S. M., Moore, S., & Walker, T. D. (2019). Barriers and facilitators to mental health help-seeking among African American youth and their families: A systematic review study. *Children and Youth Services Review, 101*, 190–200.

Robinson, W. L., Case, M. H., Whipple, C. R., Gooden, A. S., Lopez-Tamayo, R., Lambert, S. F., & Jason, L. A. (2016). Culturally grounded stress reduction and suicide prevention for

African American adolescents. *Practice Innovations, 1*(2), 117–128. https://doi.org/10.1037/pri0000020

Sheftall, A. H., & Miller, A. B. (2021). Setting a ground zero research agenda for preventing Black youth suicide. *JAMA Pediatrics, 175*(9), 890–892. https://doi.org/10.1001/jamapediatrics.2021.1112

Sheftall, A. H., Asti, L., Horowitz, L. M., Felts, A., Fontanella, C. A., Campo, J. V., & Bridge, J. A. (2016). Suicide in elementary school-aged children and early adolescents. *Pediatrics, 138*(4). https://doi.org/10.1542/peds.2016-0436

Watson Coleman, B. (2021). *H.R.1475 – Pursuing Equity in Mental Health act.* https://www.congress.gov/bill/117th-congress/senate-bill/1795

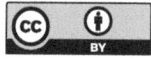

Chapter 13
Suicide and Self-Harm Prevention and Intervention in LGBTQIA+ Youth: Current Research and Future Directions

Alex Rubin, Diana M. Y. Smith, W. Cole Lawson, and Kathryn R. Fox

Youth who are lesbian, gay, bisexual, queer, and questioning their sexual identities (LGBQ+) and/or who are a gender distinct from their birth-assigned sex (i.e., transgender and gender diverse), collectively LGBTQIA+, show nearly triple the risk for self-injurious thoughts and behaviors (SITBs), including nonsuicidal self-injury, suicide ideation, and suicide attempts (Marshal et al., 2011). Unfortunately, few studies to date have rigorously tested SITB treatments in LGBTQIA+ youth. In a recent meta-analysis of all randomized controlled trials of SITB interventions, only 60/642 treatment studies reported on the LGBTQIA+ composition of the sample, and *no study* specifically focused on treatment for LGBTQIA+ youth *or* adults (Fox et al., 2020). It remains unclear if treatments designed for cisgender, heterosexual youth are similarly efficacious for LGBTQIA+ youth and regardless whether they are sufficient to reduce this heightened risk.

In this chapter, we review the state of research on SITB treatment and prevention programs for LGBTQIA+ youth. Given the high prevalence and social and emotional burden of LGBTQIA+ youth, we leverage this incomplete literature to provide steps for researchers, clinicians, and public health officials to take action *now* while we continue to build stronger evidence. We describe existing research and argue that to successfully reduce SITBs among LGBTQIA+ youth, treatment and prevention efforts should target LGBTQIA+ minority stress across individual, interpersonal, and structural levels (Chaudoir et al., 2017). Although discussed separately, each level interacts; for example, individual-level stressors (e.g., internalized stigma) are born out of the structural and interpersonal stressors that LGBTQIA+ youth face.

A. Rubin · D. M. Y. Smith · W. C. Lawson · K. R. Fox (✉)
Department of Psychology, University of Denver, Denver, CO, USA
e-mail: Alex.Rubin@du.edu; d9smith@health.ucsd.edu; William.Lawson4@va.gov; Kathryn.Fox@du.edu

© The Author(s) 2022
J. P. Ackerman, L. M. Horowitz (eds.), *Youth Suicide Prevention and Intervention*, SpringerBriefs in Psychology,
https://doi.org/10.1007/978-3-031-06127-1_13

Key Terms and Considerations

SITB rates differ across specific LGBTQIA+ identities and across intersections with birth-assigned sex, race/ethnicity, and disability. Despite these nuances, most studies on LGBTQIA+ SITBs ignore individual identities and intersections to increase sample size and power. When relevant, abbreviated acronyms will be used to represent who was included in a given study. We will state when findings support clear differences across LGBTQIA+ and intersectional identities.

Evidence for Individual Targets for Suicide Prevention

Intrapersonal attributes encompass how a person thinks, acts, and feels as they navigate their own experiences. For example, internalized stigma is the process by which some LGBTQIA+ people internally adopt the societal norm (i.e., heterosexism) and, in turn, absorb negative stereotypes and assumptions about themselves (termed internalized stigma; Meyer, 2003). A systematic review of 35 studies recently identified internalized stigma as a major risk factor for adverse mental health outcomes in LGBQ youth (Hall, 2018), providing preliminary evidence that internalized stigma likely relates to elevated SITB risk as well. Similar relationships have been observed in transgender and gender-diverse adults, with internalized transphobia associated with suicide attempts above and beyond other factors (Perez-Brumer et al., 2015).

Due to an often hostile culture, rejection sensitivity, or the tendency to readily perceive, anxiously anticipate, and avoid possible rejection, may be a risk factor for SITBs for LGBQ+ (Feinstein, 2019) and transgender and gender-diverse (Wells et al., 2020) youth. Indeed, research suggests that rejection sensitivity is associated with social anxiety, posttraumatic stress, and generalized anxiety in GB men (Cohen et al., 2016) and with suicide attempts among LGBQ+ adults (Mereish et al., 2019). LGBTQIA+ youth may also hide ("conceal") their identity to protect themselves from potential discrimination, which may cause stress, anxiety, and internalized stigma (Gleason et al., 2016). However, research linking identity concealment to psychopathology is relatively weak (Pachankis et al., 2020), and more research is needed to examine the relationship between concealment and SITBs.

Evidence for Interpersonal Targets for Suicide Prevention

Heteronormativity and binary views of gender (i.e., classification of gender into two distinct categories of man/woman) often lead to interpersonal stress and rejection for LGBTQIA+ youth by family members, friends, and peers. LGBTQIA+ youth report lower levels of family connectedness and support from teachers and other adults compared to non-LGBTQIA+youth (Eisenberg & Resnick, 2006). Bisexual and pansexual youth may face additional rejection from others in the LGBTQIA+ community and romantic partners (Feinstein, 2019). Interpersonal conflicts and rejection are consistently associated with SITBs among LGBTQIA+ individuals. For example, LGBTQIA+ young adults who died by suicide were more likely to have experienced relationship difficulties prior to death (e.g., Lyons et al., 2019).

In contrast, support from family members, friends, and communities is protective for LGBTQIA+ individuals (Puckett et al., 2019) and may play a key role in reducing SITB risk. Family connectedness and adult caring are protective against suicidal ideation and attempts among LGB youth both cross-sectionally (Eisenberg & Resnick, 2006) and longitudinally (Mustanski & Liu, 2013). Support from friends and family is negatively associated with past-year suicide attempts and ideation in transgender and gender-diverse youth (Kuper et al., 2018).

General and bias-based bullying and victimization are major stressors for many LGBTQIA+ youth (Kosciw et al., 2018). A scoping review on this topic indicates that LGBQ+ youth experience more bullying compared to their heterosexual peers and that these experiences are associated with higher rates of suicide ideation and attempts (Gower et al., 2018). Importantly, compared to other LGBTQIA+ youth, bisexual and transgender and gender-diverse youth (Gower et al., 2018; Horwitz et al., 2021) may experience particularly elevated rates of bullying and victimization. Bias-based bullying (due to LGBTQIA+ identity) may be even more harmful. Across several studies, anti-LGBQ+ discrimination was associated with higher rates of suicide attempts among youth concurrently and longitudinally (e.g., Fish et al., 2019; Mustanski and Liu, 2013). Among transgender and gender-diverse youth, violence and discrimination are especially prevalent, even compared to their cisgender LGBQ+ peers (Price-Feeney et al., 2020). Experiences of victimization and discrimination partially explain elevated SITBs in transgender and gender-diverse youth.

Evidence for Structural Targets for Suicide Prevention

The nature of most structural-level factors (e.g., city- and statewide policies, underlying cultural factors) precludes randomized controlled trials assessing their impact on SITBs. However, several studies have used large, cross-sectional, and longitudinal samples to assess the effects of policies that support LGBTQIA+ youth on mental health and SITBs. Compared to their cisgender, heterosexual peers, LGBTQIA+ youth are more likely to be homeless, with rates of homelessness ranging from 8% to 37% among this population (McCann & Brown, 2019). In addition to increasing risk for mental health difficulties and SITBs, homelessness also impacts access to mental and physical healthcare services and increases potential exposure to violence, food insecurity, and a host of other negative outcomes, each of which is disproportionately experienced by LGBTQIA+ youth (Paley, 2021). Hostile sociopolitical climates are also associated with SITBs in LGBTQIA+ youth. For example, low LGB supportiveness across the school and county level is associated with higher suicide risk (Hatzenbuehler & Pachankis, 2016).

Evidence-Based Interventions

Individual-Level Interventions

There is good news despite the many barriers to mental health equity. Interventions leveraging LGBTQIA+-affirming principles can effectively reduce internalized stigma and psychopathology. For example, interventions based on cognitive behavioral therapy (CBT) principles targeting minority-related stressors reduce internalized stigma, depression, alcohol use, and anxiety in young GB men (Pachankis et al., 2015) and LGBQ+ women (Pachankis et al., 2020). Given the strong link between internalized stigma and SITBs, these interventions may also be effective for reducing SITBs in LGBTQIA+ youth. Briefly, given evidence that interventions targeting psychopathology and SITBs show similar efficacy (Fox et al., 2020), interventions targeting psychopathology may also reduce SITBs in LGBTQIA+ youth. In light of the unique stressors faced by LGBTQIA+ youth, these treatments should be modified to incorporate modules and frameworks that incorporate these unique experiences (see Smithee et al., 2019). At least one uncontrolled study provides preliminary efficacy for this approach (Lucassen et al., 2015).

Interpersonal-Level Interventions

Interventions designed to bolster familial support and acceptance of LGBTQIA+ children may help to reduce SITBs. In a small ($n = 10$), uncontrolled study, an adapted model of attachment-based family therapy for LGBQ+ youth significantly reduced suicidal ideation (Diamond et al., 2012). Other interventions targeting parents of LGBTQIA+ youth that have shown potential include an educational film (Huebner et al., 2013), interactive online modules (Goodman & Israel, 2020), and expressive writing (Abreu & Kenny, 2017). As reviewed by Chaudoir et al. (2017), other interpersonal-level interventions seek to (1) increase contact and empathy with LGBQ+ people, (2) teach caregivers, health providers, teachers, and peers to reduce LGBQ+-based discrimination, and (3) increase LGBQ+-affirming behaviors. Each of these intervention targets demonstrates preliminary support. Across both experimental and correlational studies, intergroup contact— across teachers, medical providers, and students—increases positive attitudes and empathy toward LGBTQIA+ youth (Smith et al., 2009), and interventions have increased LGB-affirming behaviors and decreased rejection (Chaudoir et al., 2017). Future research is needed to test whether these interventions can reduce LGBTQIA+ discrimination long term and whether they lead to decreases in SITBs among LGBTQIA+ youth.

Structural-Level Interventions

Improved school climates and supportive environments across city and state levels also reduce SITBs across LGBTQIA+ youth (Gleason et al., 2016). Two factors may be key: anti-bullying policies including LGBTQIA+ youth as a protected group and gay/gender-straight alliances (GSAs). At the school and district level, anti-bullying policies are associated with reduced risk of suicide attempts (Hatzenbuehler & Keyes, 2013). The benefits of GSAs are also widely documented; schools with GSAs have fewer suicide attempts (Poteat et al., 2013), and students experience less homophobic victimization, fear for their safety, and homophobic remarks (Marx & Kettrey, 2016). Of note, several confounding factors co-occur with the presence of a GSA (e.g., larger schools, more experienced teachers; Baams et al., 2018). Additionally, state-level policies banning insurance policies from gender-based discrimination were associated with decreased suicidality in transgender and gender-diverse people (McDowell et al., 2020). Finally, indicating the importance of federal, LGBTQIA+-affirming policies, same-sex marriage policies have been associated with an estimated 134,446 fewer suicide attempts per year among high school students, with this effect driven by LGBQ+ students (Raifman et al., 2017).

Conclusions and Recommendations

Interventions that reduce minority stressors and increase coping skills in the context of minority stress are most effective. Although large randomized controlled trials using diverse samples of LGBTQIA+ youth are needed, interventions across levels and targets will likely result in the largest reductions in SITBs. In addition to inter- and intrapersonal-level interventions, we argue that major structural changes are needed to meaningfully reduce elevated risk for SITBs.

Policy Makers and Community Leaders

LGBTQIA+ inclusive and protective policies decrease SITBs in LGBTQIA+ youth. Continued creation and enforcement of LGBTQIA+-affirming, supportive, and protective policies are needed to reduce SITB risk in LGBTQIA+ youth. For example, federal and state-level laws should explicitly include sexual orientation and gender identity in laws protecting against discrimination and harassment in schools, housing, and the workplace; healthcare policies should explicitly prohibit discrimination based on gender and sexual identities.

Clinicians

Education for clinicians should include LGBTQIA+-affirming language and practices to reduce stigma, harassment, and insufficient care. This will decrease barriers and increase use of lifesaving physical and mental healthcare for LGBTQIA+ youth. Moreover, access to gender-affirming, including medical transition, services for transgender and gender-diverse individuals seeking such services decreases risk for SITBs (Bauer et al., 2015). Training programs and licensure exams should ensure that clinicians are knowledgeable of these services (e.g., local providers, requirements, structural barriers) and should teach clinicians to direct transgender and gender-diverse clients to gender-affirming care as desired while recognizing that individuals' needs and desires will differ.

Researchers

Increased emphasis must be placed on recruiting diverse and representative samples; for too long, majority-white samples have remained the norm. Innovative methods are needed to engage racially diverse LGBTQIA+ youth and families, and researchers should aim for sufficient sample size for disaggregation of intersectional identity subgroups. Randomized controlled trials including active control groups and SITB outcomes in studies testing LGBTQIA+ interventions are also needed. When studying structural-level impacts on SITBs, quasi-experimental designs during major policy changes (e.g., after legalization of same-sex marriage) may allow for a more thorough investigation of potential confounding factors, compared to the existing, largely cross-sectional literature.

References

Abreu, R. L., & Kenny, M. C. (2017). Cyberbullying and LGBTQ youth: A systematic literature review and recommendations for prevention and intervention. *Journal of Child & Adolescent Trauma, 11*(1), 81–97. https://doi.org/10.1007/s40653-017-0175-7

Baams, L., Pollitt, A. M., Laub, C., & Russell, S. T. (2018). Characteristics of schools with and without Gay-Straight Alliances. *Applied Developmental Science, 24*(4), 1–6. https://doi.org/10.1080/10888691.2018.1510778

Bauer, G. R., Scheim, A. I., Pyne, J., Travers, R., & Hammond, R. (2015). Intervenable factors associated with suicide risk in transgender persons: A respondent driven sampling study in Ontario, Canada. *BMC Public Health, 15*(1), 525. https://doi.org/10.1186/s12889-015-1867-2

Chaudoir, S. R., Wang, K., & Pachankis, J. E. (2017). What reduces sexual minority stress? A review of the intervention "Toolkit". *Journal of Social Issues, 73*(3), 586–617. https://doi.org/10.1111/josi.12233

Cohen, J. M., Feinstein, B. A., Rodriguez-Seijas, C., Taylor, C. B., & Newman, M. G. (2016). Rejection sensitivity as a transdiagnostic risk factor for internalizing psychopathology among gay and bisexual men. *Psychology of Sexual Orientation and Gender Diversity, 3*(3), 259–264. https://doi.org/10.1037/sgd0000170

Diamond, G. M., Diamond, G. S., Levy, S., Closs, C., Ladipo, T., & Siqueland, L. (2012). Attachment-based family therapy for suicidal lesbian, gay, and bisexual adolescents: A treatment development study and open trial with preliminary findings. *Psychotherapy, 49*(1), 62–71. https://doi.org/10.1037/a0026247

Eisenberg, M. E., & Resnick, M. D. (2006). Suicidality among gay, lesbian and bisexual youth: The role of protective factors. *Journal of Adolescent Health, 39*(5), 662–668. https://doi.org/10.1016/j.jadohealth.2006.04.024

Feinstein, B. A. (2019). The rejection sensitivity model as a framework for understanding sexual minority mental health. *Archives of Sexual Behavior.* https://doi.org/10.1007/s10508-019-1428-3

Fish, J. N., Rice, C. E., Lanza, S. T., & Russell, S. T. (2019). Is young adulthood a critical period for suicidal behavior among sexual minorities? Results from a US national sample. *Prevention Science, 20*(3), 353–365. https://doi.org/10.1007/s11121-018-0878-5

Fox, K. R., Huang, X., Guzmán, E. M., Funsch, K. M., Cha, C. B., Ribeiro, J. D., & Franklin, J. C. (2020). Interventions for suicide and self-injury: A meta-analysis of randomized controlled trials across nearly 50 years of research. *Psychological Bulletin, 146,* 1117–1145. https://doi.org/10.1037/bul0000305

Gleason, H. A., Livingston, N. A., Peters, M. M., Oost, K. M., Reely, E., & Cochran, B. N. (2016). Effects of state nondiscrimination laws on transgender and gender-nonconforming individuals' perceived community stigma and mental health. *Journal of Gay & Lesbian Mental Health, 20*(4), 350–362. https://doi.org/10.1080/19359705.2016.1207582

Goodman, J. A., & Israel, T. (2020). An online intervention to promote predictors of supportive parenting for sexual minority youth. *Journal of Family Psychology, 34*(1), 90–100. https://doi.org/10.1037/fam0000614

Gower, A. L., Rider, G. N., McMorris, B. J., & Eisenberg, M. E. (2018). Bullying victimization among LGBTQ youth: Current and future directions. *Current Sexual Health Reports, 10*(4), 246–254. https://doi.org/10.1007/s11930-018-0169-y

Hall, W. J. (2018). Psychosocial risk and protective factors for depression among lesbian, gay, bisexual, and queer youth: A systematic review. *Journal of Homosexuality, 65*(3), 263–316. https://doi.org/10.1080/00918369.2017.1317467

Hatzenbuehler, M. L., & Keyes, K. M. (2013). Inclusive anti-bullying policies and reduced risk of suicide attempts in lesbian and gay youth. *Journal of Adolescent Health, 53*(1), S21–S26. https://doi.org/10.1016/j.jadohealth.2012.08.010

Hatzenbuehler, M. L., & Pachankis, J. E. (2016). Stigma and minority stress as social determinants of health among lesbian, gay, bisexual, and transgender youth. *Pediatric Clinics of North America, 63*(6), 985–997. https://doi.org/10.1016/j.pcl.2016.07.003

Horwitz, A. G., Grupp-Phelan, J., Brent, D., Barney, B. J., Casper, T. C., Berona, J., Chernick, L. S., Shenoi, R., Cwik, M., King, C. A., & Pediatric Emergency Care Applied Research Network. (2021). Risk and protective factors for suicide among sexual minority youth seeking emergency medical services. *Journal of Affective Disorders, 279,* 274–281. https://doi.org/10.1016/j.jad.2020.10.015

Huebner, D. M., Rullo, J. E., Thoma, B. C., McGarrity, L., & Mackenzie, J. (2013). Piloting lead with love: A film-based intervention to improve parents' responses to their lesbian, gay, and bisexual children. *The Journal of Primary Prevention, 34*(5), 359–369. https://doi.org/10.1007/s10935-013-0319-y

Kosciw, J. G., Greytak, E. A., Zongrone, A. D., Clark, C. M., & Truong, N. L. (2018). *The 2017 National School Climate Survey: The experiences of lesbian, gay, bisexual, transgender, and queer youth in our nation's schools.* New York: GLSEN.

Kuper, L. E., Adams, N., & Mustanski, B. S. (2018). Exploring cross-sectional predictors of suicide ideation, attempt, and risk in a large online sample of transgender and gender nonconforming youth and young adults. *LGBT Health, 5*(7), 391–400. https://doi.org/10.1089/lgbt.2017.0259

Lucassen, M. F. G., Merry, S. N., Hatcher, S., & Frampton, C. M. A. (2015). Rainbow SPARX: A novel approach to addressing depression in sexual minority youth. *Cognitive and Behavioral Practice, 22*(2), 203–216. https://doi.org/10.1016/j.cbpra.2013.12.008

Lyons, B. H., Walters, M. L., Jack, S. P. D., Petrosky, E., Blair, J. M., & Ivey-Stephenson, A. Z. (2019). Suicides among lesbian and gay male individuals: Findings from the national violent death reporting system. *American Journal of Preventive Medicine, 56*(4), 512–521. https://doi.org/10.1016/j.amepre.2018.11.012

Marshal, M. P., Dietz, L. J., Friedman, M. S., Stall, R., Smith, H., McGinley, J., Thoma, B. C., Murray, P. J., D'Augelli, A., & Brent, D. A. (2011). Suicidality and depression disparities between sexual minority and heterosexual youth: A meta-analytic review. *The Journal of Adolescent Health, 49*(2), 115–123. https://doi.org/10.1016/j.jadohealth.2011.02.005

Marx, R. A., & Kettrey, H. H. (2016). Gay-straight alliances are associated with lower levels of school-based victimization of LGBTQIA+ youth: A systematic review and meta-analysis. *Journal of Youth and Adolescence, 45*(7), 1269–1282. https://doi.org/10.1007/s10964-016-0501-7

McCann, E., & Brown, M. (2019). Homelessness among youth who identify as LGBTQIA+: A systematic review. *Journal of Clinical Nursing, 28*(11–12), 2061–2072. https://doi.org/10.1111/jocn.14818

McDowell, A., Raifman, J., Progovac, A. M., & Rose, S. (2020). Association of nondiscrimination policies with mental health among gender minority individuals. *JAMA Psychiatry, 77*(9), 952–958. https://doi.org/10.1001/jamapsychiatry.2020.0770

Mereish, E. H., Peters, J. R., & Yen, S. (2019). Minority stress and relational mechanisms of suicide among sexual minorities: Subgroup differences in the associations between heterosexist victimization, shame, rejection sensitivity, and suicide risk. *Suicide & Life-Threatening Behavior, 49*(2), 547–560. https://doi.org/10.1111/sltb.12458

Meyer, I. H. (2003). Prejudice, social stress, and mental health in lesbian, gay, and bisexual populations: Conceptual issues and research evidence. *Psychological Bulletin, 129*(5), 674–697. https://doi.org/10.1037/0033-2909.129.5.674

Mustanski, B., & Liu, R. T. (2013). A longitudinal study of predictors of suicide attempts among lesbian, gay, bisexual, and transgender youth. *Archives of Sexual Behavior, 42*(3), 437–448. https://doi.org/10.1007/s10508-012-0013-9

Pachankis, J. E., Hatzenbuehler, M. L., Rendina, H. J., Safren, S. A., & Parsons, J. T. (2015). LGB-affirmative cognitive-behavioral therapy for young adult gay and bisexual men: A randomized controlled trial of a transdiagnostic minority stress approach. *Journal of Consulting and Clinical Psychology, 83*(5), 875–889. https://doi.org/10.1037/ccp0000037

Pachankis, J. E., McConocha, E. M., Clark, K. A., Wang, K., Behari, K., Fetzner, B. K., Brisbin, C. D., Scheer, J. R., & Lehavot, K. (2020). A transdiagnostic minority stress intervention for gender diverse sexual minority women's depression, anxiety, and unhealthy alcohol use: A randomized controlled trial. *Journal of Consulting and Clinical Psychology, 88*(7), 613–630. https://doi.org/10.1037/ccp0000508

Paley, A. (2021). *National survey on LGBTQ youth mental health.* https://www.thetrevorproject.org/wp-content/uploads/2021/05/The-Trevor-Project-National-Survey-Results-2021.pdf

Perez-Brumer, A., Hatzenbuehler, M. L., Oldenburg, C. E., & Bockting, W. (2015). Individual- and structural-level risk factors for suicide attempts among transgender adults. *Behavioral Medicine, 41*(3), 164–171. https://doi.org/10.1080/08964289.2015.1028322

Poteat, V. P., Sinclair, K. O., DiGiovanni, C. D., Koenig, B. W., & Russell, S. T. (2013). Gay–straight alliances are associated with student health: A multischool comparison of LGBTQ and heterosexual youth. *Journal of Research on Adolescence, 23*(2), 319–330. https://doi.org/10.1111/j.1532-7795.2012.00832.x

Price-Feeney, M., Green, A. E., & Dorison, S. (2020). Understanding the mental health of transgender and nonbinary youth. *Journal of Adolescent Health, 66*(6), 684–690. https://doi.org/10.1016/j.jadohealth.2019.11.314

Puckett, J. A., Matsuno, E., Dyar, C., Mustanski, B., & Newcomb, M. E. (2019). Mental health and resilience in transgender individuals: What type of support makes a difference? *Journal of Family Psychology, 33*(8), 954–964. https://doi.org/10.1037/fam0000561

Raifman, J., Moscoe, E., Austin, S. B., & McConnell, M. (2017). Difference-in-differences analysis of the association between state same-sex marriage policies and adolescent suicide attempts. *JAMA Pediatrics, 171*(4), 350–356. https://doi.org/10.1001/jamapediatrics.2016.4529

Smith, S. J., Axelton, A. M., & Saucier, D. A. (2009). The effects of contact on sexual prejudice: A meta-analysis. *Sex Roles, 61*(3), 178–191. https://doi.org/10.1007/s11199-009-9627-3

Smithee, L. C., Sumner, B. W., & Bean, R. A. (2019). Non-suicidal self-injury among sexual minority youth: An etiological and treatment overview. *Children and Youth Services Review, 96*, 212–219. https://doi.org/10.1016/j.childyouth.2018.11.055

Wells, T. T., Tucker, R. P., & Kraines, M. A. (2020). Extending a rejection sensitivity model to suicidal thoughts and behaviors in sexual minority groups and to transgender mental health. *Archives of Sexual Behavior, 49*(7), 2291–2294. https://doi.org/10.1007/s10508-019-01596-8

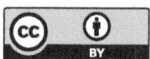

Chapter 14
Preventing Suicide in Youth with Intellectual and Neurodevelopmental Disorders: Lessons Learned and Policy Recommendations

Katie Johanning-Gray, Pankhuree Vandana, Jacqueline Wynn, and Jane Hamel-Lambert

Suicidality in Intellectual and Neurodevelopmental Disabilities

Autism spectrum disorder (ASD) is a neurodevelopmental disorder characterized by social communication deficits and the presence of repetitive and restricted behaviors. Based on tracking of 8-year-old children within 11 communities in the USA, 1 in 54 children was identified with ASD in 2016 by the CDC's Autism and Developmental Disabilities Monitoring (ADDM) Network (Maenner et al., 2020). Mayes et al. (2013) found that 14% of youth with ASD were endorsed by mothers as experiencing suicidal thoughts and behaviors whereas only 0.5% of neurotypical children were rated by mothers as having these same concerns. Baer et al. (2020) reported that 41.8% of parents registered with the Interactive Autism Network (IAN) noted that their child or dependent adult (25 years or younger) had displayed suicidal behaviors. Furthermore, the most commonly reported age of onset for both passive and active suicidal ideation was 8 years old or younger. Children as young as 5 years old were reported by their parents as having tried to end their life. Within the IAN sample, 3.5% had attempted suicide.

Several ASD symptoms overlap with known suicide risk factors. Further, ASD is associated with many comorbid mental health conditions. Research has explored the influence of impaired social communication and cognitive flexibility, social isolation, bullying, high rates of psychiatric comorbidities (e.g., depression, anxiety, ADHD, trauma), impulsivity, deficits in understanding the temporal sequencing and durability of events, masking/camouflaging, and alexithymia on suicidal behavior

K. Johanning-Gray (✉) · P. Vandana · J. Wynn · J. Hamel-Lambert
Nationwide Children's Hospital, Columbus, OH, USA

The Ohio State University, Columbus, OH, USA
e-mail: Katie.Johanning-Gray@nationwidechildrens.org;
Pankhuree.Vandana@nationwidechildrens.org;
Jacquie.Wynn@nationwidechildrens.org; Jane.Hamel-Lambert@nationwidechildrens.org

© The Author(s) 2022
J. P. Ackerman, L. M. Horowitz (eds.), *Youth Suicide Prevention and Intervention*, SpringerBriefs in Psychology,
https://doi.org/10.1007/978-3-031-06127-1_14

(Baer et al., 2020; Cassidy, et al., 2020; Joshi et al., 2010; Mayes et al., 2013; Richa, et al., 2014; Storch et al., 2013). Conversely, the psychiatric hospitalization of youth due to their suicidal behavior may lead to the identification of intellectual and neurodevelopmental disorders (INDs) by their treatment team. In some medical settings, consults for neurodevelopmental evaluations of psychiatrically hospitalized youth may be completed to aide in establishing immediate safety and treatment planning for at-risk youth.

Intellectual disability (ID), which often accompanies ASD, does not have a protective effect against suicide. Horowitz et al. (2018) studied children between the ages of 10 and 18 with ASD, a quarter of whom had mild ID. They found that 63% of parents indicated that their child "talks about death or suicide" for a "period lasting several days." "Frequent periods" of talking about death or suicide were reported in 22% of the sample. Their analyses further explored rates of suicidal ideation among children within three ranges of intellectual ability reporting 25.4% in those with an IQ above 85, 20% in those with IQ below 70, and 15.4% for those with IQs between 70 and 85.

Another source of data that sheds light on the prevalence of suicide attempts and deaths is the Ohio Department of Developmental Disabilities (ODODD) which tracks these outcomes among its more than 95,000 consumers aged 10 to 60. From 2015 through 2019, ODODD reported that 15 individuals with developmental disabilities died by suicide, 8 of whom had a diagnosis of ASD. Of these eight individuals, all were male, 50% were 21 or younger, and 25% had ID. Between 2012 and 2019, there were 182 suicide attempts. Of those making attempts, 40% did not have an intellectual disability, 35% had mild ID, 6% had moderate ID, and 0.6% had severe ID; 56% of these consumers had at least one comorbid mental health condition, and 44% had made a prior attempt (Internal ODODD data retrieved 2020). These findings, pulled from a large population data set, provide strong foundational information about suicidality in persons with INDs. It corroborates the occurrence of suicide attempts in children as young as age 10, with a preponderance of reported attempts and deaths by suicide occurring in individuals who are under the age of 30.

Collectively, these data substantiate the urgent need to ensure universal suicide screening inclusive of children and adolescents with INDs. However, there are few evidence-based tools available to researchers and clinicians that can be used with individuals with INDs. Frequently, individuals with INDs are excluded from research studies despite the possibility of inclusion with minimal adaptation (Feldman et al., 2014). There are adverse consequences to excluding individuals with INDs from research studies designed to establish the effectiveness of instruments and intervention particularly as it relates to suicide risk. The generalizability of current tools and interventions which have been validated on neurotypical samples is unknown, leaving parents and providers relying on observation and intuition, rather than science. Excluding individuals with ID from research efforts is problematic and potentially harmful despite the well-intended goal of preventing harm among those with ID. Although including individuals with neurodevelopmental disabilities in research requires heightened engagement, creativity, and patience, doing so results in findings and recommended practices that are generalizable to a broader spectrum of youth (Carlson, 2013).

Lessons Learned in Suicide Prevention in Youth with INDs

Due to the lack of validated suicide screening tools and interventions, clinical providers often struggle with how to appropriately complete these essential responsibilities with patients with INDs. This section outlines suicide prevention efforts for individuals with INDs conducted at Nationwide Children's Hospital (NCH), a large pediatric hospital in the Midwest. It can serve as a road map for other healthcare organizations and further the conversation regarding best practices in suicide prevention for youth with INDs. One gap identified with respect to suicide prevention was the consistent use of a validated suicide risk screening tool. Across numerous internal planning discussions regarding the design of suicide prevention policies at NCH, the validity of conducting universal screening with the Ask Suicide-Screening Questions (ASQ; Horowitz et al., 2012) tool for children presenting for either neurodevelopmental assessment or treatment for ASD was debated. Decisions were made at the unit level to design protocols that best matched their service line. At the NCH Child Development Center, a center which focuses on the assessment of ASD and other INDs as well as treatment for individuals with INDs, and NCH Center for Autism Spectrum Disorder, which focuses on treatment for youth with ASD, we have implemented broad suicide screening of all patients 10 years old and above. Exceptions to this screening may be made when the clinician determines that the screening would be developmentally inappropriate (e.g., a verbal IQ lower than 70). Our experiences have confirmed the value of suicide prevention policies that are inclusive of children with ASD and other INDs. Universal suicide screening was launched for children presenting to these NCH centers in July 2019. Through the second week of February 2021, 1410 ASQs were completed at the Child Development Center; approximately 15.2% had a positive screen (a "yes" to any of four initial suicide-specific questions), and 0.57% had a positive screen on Question 5, asking if the child had present thoughts of killing themselves following a positive response to one of the first four items. At the NCH Center for Autism Spectrum Disorder outpatient treatment program, 400 ASQs were completed during the same time period; approximately 35.7% had a positive screen, and 3.0% were positive on Question 5 (Internal NCH data retrieved on Feb. 17, 2021).

Considerations in Screening, Risk Assessment, and Safety Planning: Illustrative Vignettes

Enhanced screening, risk assessment, and safety planning have become the standard of care across the behavioral health service line at NCH over the several years including for youth with ASD and other INDs. Use of a program-wide screener (e.g., ASQ) for suicidal thoughts and behaviors has been critical in identifying individuals at risk for suicidal behaviors and engaging in appropriate safety planning for them. Along with the utility of the ASQ, we have found through continuous quality improvement efforts that clinical best practices have emerged. We share some of these cases to highlight the nuances in assessment and management of suicidality as well as recommendations for safe and effective care with this population.

Several consistent observations have guided adaptations. As we have administered the ASQ to children with INDs, it has become apparent that some patients struggle with understanding timeframes such as "within the past few weeks" and "in the past week" on the ASQ. In the case of a 12-year-old male diagnosed with ASD, without language and intellectual delays, and ADHD receiving psychiatric care at our clinic, when asked if he had thoughts of killing himself in the last week, he responded "yes." Furthermore, when asked if he had ever tried to kill himself, he responded "yes" and then stated that the attempt had occurred at school during the past week. His caregivers expressed shock at this revelation as no recent incident report was sent by school; however, they described similar past incidents that had been reported to them by school staff. Collateral information from the school clarified that such an incident had occurred several months ago and the school team had verbally de-escalated the patient to safety. This case highlights that children within this population may struggle with the abstract concept of time; in response, clinicians have offered specific dates to help anchor the timeline for patients in these situations.

We have also encountered other cases at our clinic where patients' understanding of the intent of the ASQ questions limited their utility. In another case, a 14-year-old male who presented to our clinic for evaluation of ASD, and who was later diagnosed with ASD without language or intellectual delays, struggled with the phrase "better off" in Question 2 ("In the past few weeks, have you felt that you or your family would be better off if you were dead?") of the ASQ. In response to the question, he stated, "what do you mean 'off,' like turning a computer 'off?'." The clinician again attempted to ask the question verbatim, and the patient continued to be confused. Finally, the clinician rephrased the question by replacing "better off" with "happier," the patient seemed to understand the meaning of the question at that point, and the patient was able to provide an answer.

Recommendations for Screening, Risk Assessment, and Safety Planning

We offer several recommendations to address these challenges. As the phrasing of screening questions appears to be understood by most individuals with INDs, clinicians should continue to ask screening questions verbatim, consistent with initial validation studies and administration guidance (see Mournet et al., this volume). However, in some cases it will become evident that the patient does not understand the intent of the question. In those cases, clinicians should not abandon the screening, but rather, they should be prepared to modify the question(s) to complete a screening of the patient while assessing for adequate comprehension of each question's intended meaning.

When assessing for suicidality in children with ASD and ID, the heterogeneity of self-injurious behaviors must also be considered. Hunsche et al. (2020) highlight that self-injurious behavior in children with ASD does not always indicate the presence of suicidal intent. In our practice at the Child Development Center and Center for Autism Spectrum Disorder, visual supports have proven useful in clarifying the underlying function and intent of the self-injurious behaviors. Additionally, these visual supports benefit safety planning as they allow for strong individualization of the safety plan and collaborative patient engagement in the safety planning process.

The case of "Sarah," a 13-year-old female, illustrates the use of visuals and assessment of self-injurious behaviors. Sarah is diagnosed with mild ID and has a history of two previous self-aborted suicide attempts; she presented for treatment of panic attacks, recurrent suicidal ideation, and non-suicidal self-injurious behaviors (NSSIB). She had a history of multiple hospitalizations in the past due to her complex clinical presentation. Sarah struggled to verbally report intent behind NSSIB as compared to suicidal ideation. Clinicians utilized concrete visual supports to assess her motivation behind the self-injurious behaviors, including identifying a graveyard as a symbol to depict end of life when clarifying suicidal intent. From the beginning, the safety plan was identified as belonging to Sarah, so she had choice and control of its content. She was able to choose her preferred color and font for the text of the plan. Color associations and thermometers previously learned in cognitive behavioral therapy to describe emotions were included. Pictures Sarah chose from Google Images of the precursor behaviors were also placed in the "Warning Signs" section along with a few descriptive words and pictures she chose to illustrate preferred activities. Personal interests were also included in her plan. Additionally, due to Sarah's struggles with self-awareness and decreased self-monitoring capacity, specific need for close adult supervision and monitoring was discussed with caregivers. As the safety plan is considered to be a "living document," it continued to be modified during treatment. As other triggers, drivers for suicidal behavior, and coping strategies were identified in later visits, they were incorporated in her plan. In order to fully include individuals with INDs in the process of screening, assessment, and safety planning, visual supports are useful. Figure 14.1 provides examples of how visual supports can be utilized.

There are instances when a patient's level of cognitive ability interferes with understanding the questions as intended and the ASQ is deemed to be "developmentally inappropriate." For individuals with INDs who are unable to complete the ASQ or other suicide risk screeners, alternative safety screening methods are recommended. For example, individuals with less impaired communication may be able to engage in a conversation with the clinician which will allow for clarification and frequent perception checking. Individuals with more impaired communication abilities may take part in a conversation with the clinician with an informed caregiver who is familiar with their language abilities as part of the conversation.

Warning Signs:

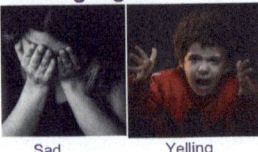

Sad   Yelling

Things I Can Do to Cope:

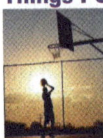 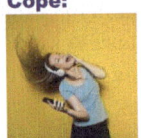

Play Basketball   Listen to Music

People or Things to Distract Me:

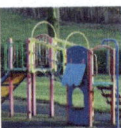 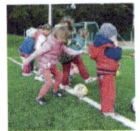

Playground   Play Soccer with Joe

People I can Ask for Help From:

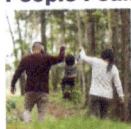

Dad and Maria

Warning Signs At School:

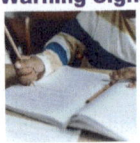 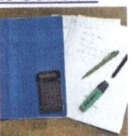

Having to Write   Math Class

Things I can Do to Cope At School:

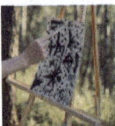 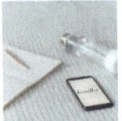

Paint   Take Deep Breaths

Things to Distract Me At School:

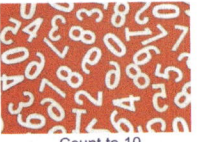 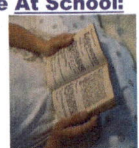

Count to 10   Read a Book

Adult at School I can Ask for Help:

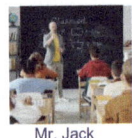 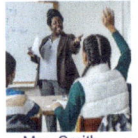

Mr. Jack   Mrs. Smith

Who I Can Call for Help:
Mom XXX-XXX-XXXX
Dr. Alex XXX-XXX-XXXX
911
County Crisis Line: XXX-XXX-XXXX
Text: 741-741

Two Things That Are Very Important to Me and Worth Living For:

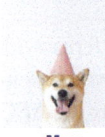 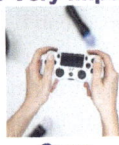

Max   **Game**

Fig. 14.1 Examples of a safety plan utilizing visual cues (pictures). A safety plan should be created in collaboration with the patient and can be modified during treatment. (pexels.com)

Future Directions and Policy Implications

Additional research is needed to validate existing tools and provide clinical guidance in the pediatric IND populations. The vignettes and discussion illustrate how two centers at NCH used clinical discretion and creativity to meaningfully adapt existing tools for the pediatric IND populations. More guidance in this area will be important for clinicians and families.

There are several ways in which work in this area can be advanced. In order to create appropriate tools for this population, funding agencies should support the inclusion of individuals with INDs in population-based research on suicide prevention. Research should be conducted to identify needed modifications to screening processes, to assess the effectiveness of safety planning, and to clarify other necessary treatment components to serve the unique needs of patients with suicidality and ASD/INDs. Licensing and accrediting bodies should consider mandating universal screening for youth age 10 and up. It is further recommended that the credentialing and licensing authorities for the various health professions review and consider requiring, or otherwise prioritizing, training on suicide prevention, risk assessment, and safety planning for specialty populations, including ASD/INDs. As The Joint Commission (2016) requirement has pushed institutions to incorporate standardized implementation of screening measures, institutions like NCH have recognized the need for formal training on assessment and management of suicidality in this high-risk population, with special focus on implementation of existing tools using a developmental approach.

References

Baer, B. L., Law, J. K., Kalb, L., Marvin, A. F., Vasa, R. A., Wilcox, H. C., & Lipkin, P. H. (2020). *Suicidal ideation and behaviors in children, youth, and young adults with autism spectrum Disorder (ASD): Rates and outcomes based on parent-report of 92 individuals with ASD*. International Society for Autism Research Annual Meeting.

Carlson, L. (2013). Research ethics and intellectual disability: Broadening the debates. *The Yale Journal of Biology and Medicine, 86*(3), 303.

Cassidy, S. A., Gould, K., Townsend, E., Pelton, M., Robertson, A. E., & Rodgers, J. (2020). Is Camouflaging autistic traits associated with suicidal thoughts and behaviours? Expanding the interpersonal psychological theory of suicide in an undergraduate student sample. *Journal of Autism and Developmental Disorders, 50*(10), 3638–3648. https://doi.org/10.1007/s10803-019-04323-3

CDC. Web-based Injury Statistics Query and Reporting System (WISQARS). (2020) Atlanta, GA: National Center for Injury Prevention and Control. https://www.cdc.gov/injury/wisqars/index.html

Feldman, M. A., Bosett, J., Collet, C., & Burnham-Riosa, P. (2014). Where are persons with intellectual disabilities in medical research? A survey of published clinical trials. *Journal of Intellectual Disability Research, 58*(9), 800–809. https://doi.org/10.1111/jir.12091

Horowitz, L. M., Bridge, J. A., Teach, S. J., Ballard, E., Klima, J., Rosenstein, D. L., Wharff, E. A., Ginnis, K., Cannon, E., Joshi, P., & Pao, M. (2012). Ask suicide-screening questions (ASQ): A brief instrument for the pediatric emergency department. *Archives of Pediatrics & Adolescent Medicine, 166*(12), 1170–1176. https://doi.org/10.1001/archpediatrics.2012.1276

Horowitz, L. M., Thurm, A., Farmer, C., Mazefsky, C., Lanzillo, E., Bridge, J. A., Greenbaum, R., Pao, M., Siegel, M., & Autism and Developmental Disorders Inpatient Research Collaborative (ADDIRC). (2018). Talking about death or suicide: Prevalence and clinical correlates in youth with autism spectrum disorder in the psychiatric inpatient setting. *Journal of Autism and Developmental Disorders, 48*(11), 3702–3710. https://doi.org/10.1007/s10803-017-3180-7

Hunsche, M. C., Saqui, S., Mirenda, P., Zaidman-Zait, A., Bennett, T., Duku, E., Elsabbagh, M., Georgiades, S., Smith, I. M., Szatmari, P., Ungar, W. J., Vaillancourt, T., Waddell, C., Zwaigenbaum, L., & Kerns, C. M. (2020). Parent-reported rates and clinical correlates of suicidality in children with autism spectrum disorder: A longitudinal study. *Journal of Autism and Developmental Disorders, 50*(10), 3496–3509. https://doi.org/10.1007/s10803-020-04373-y

Joshi, G., Petty, C., Wozniak, J., Henin, A., Fried, R., Galdo, M., Kotarski, M., Walls, S., & Biederman, J. (2010). The heavy burden of psychiatric comorbidity in youth with autism spectrum disorders: A large comparative study of a psychiatrically referred population. *Journal of Autism and Developmental Disorders, 40*(11), 1361–1370. https://doi.org/10.1007/s10803-010-0996-9

Maenner, M. J., Shaw, K. A., & Baio, J. (2020). Prevalence of autism spectrum disorder among children aged 8 years—Autism and developmental disabilities monitoring network, 11 sites, United States, 2016. *MMWR Surveillance Summaries, 69*(4), 1–12.

Mayes, S. D., Gorman, A. A., Hillwig-Garcia, J., & Syed, E. (2013). Suicide ideation and attempts in children with autism. *Research in Autism Spectrum Disorders, 7*(1), 109–119.

Richa, S., Fahed, M., Khoury, E., & Mishara, B. (2014). Suicide in autism spectrum disorders. *Archives of Suicide Research, 18*(4), 327–339. https://doi.org/10.1080/13811118.2013.824834

Storch, E. A., Sulkowski, M. L., Nadeau, J., Lewin, A. B., Arnold, E. B., Mutch, P. J., Jones, A. M., & Murphy, T. K. (2013). The phenomenology and clinical correlates of suicidal thoughts and behaviors in youth with autism spectrum disorders. *Journal of Autism and Developmental Disorders, 43*(10), 2450–2459. https://doi.org/10.1007/s10803-013-1795-x.

The Joint Commission. (2016). *2016 National Patient Safety Goals*. https://www.jointcommission.org/standards_information/npsgs.aspx

Zablotsky, B., Black, L. I., & Blumberg, S. J. (2017). *Estimated prevalence of children with diagnosed developmental disabilities in the United States, 2014–2016* (NCHS Data Brief, no 291). National Center for Health Statistics.

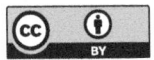

Part V
Improving Quality of Suicide Care Across Systems

Chapter 15
Investing in Suicide Prevention: Zero Suicide in a Pediatric System of Care

Glenn V. Thomas, Meredith R. Chapman, and Julie Goldstein Grumet

Youth suicide continues to be of significant concern, with the number of youth presenting for suicidal thoughts and behaviors to pediatric hospitals across the nation doubling between 2008 and 2015 (Plemmons et al., 2018). Many youth treated in emergency settings do not receive follow-up care, and even those who do fail to show improved outcomes (Asarnow et al., 2011). When risk for suicide is detected, the current standard of care is to hospitalize youth deemed to be at imminent risk. This remains the case despite an absence of randomized controlled trials demonstrating this approach alone saves lives (Kennard et al., 2019; Goldman-Mellor et al., 2021). Inpatient hospitalization temporarily protects suicidal patients from engaging in self-harm by restricting access to lethal means. However, most patients receive little or no suicide-specific treatment, and risk for suicidal behavior remains extremely high in the month after discharge (Chung et al., 2019). Furthermore, most hospitalized adolescents who attempt suicide receive limited follow-up care (Doupnik et al., 2020; Spirito et al., 2011). Rates of noncompliance with first appointments post-hospitalization have been reported to be as high as 42%, and in at least one study of adolescent suicide attempters, 25% never attended a single follow-up appointment (Burns et al., 2008; National Action Alliance for Suicide Prevention, 2017). This is concerning as follow-up mental healthcare within 7 days of discharge has been associated with a decreased risk of suicide (Fontanella et al.,

G. V. Thomas (✉) · M. R. Chapman
Big Lots Behavioral Health Services, Nationwide Children's Hospital, Columbus, OH, USA

Department of Psychiatry & Behavioral Health, The Ohio State University College of Medicine, Columbus, OH, USA
e-mail: Glenn.Thomas@nationwidechildrens.org;
Meredith.Chapman@nationwidechildrens.org

J. G. Grumet
Zero Suicide Institute, Education Development Center, Waltham, MA, USA
e-mail: JGoldstein@edc.org

© The Author(s) 2022
J. P. Ackerman, L. M. Horowitz (eds.), *Youth Suicide Prevention and Intervention*, SpringerBriefs in Psychology,
https://doi.org/10.1007/978-3-031-06127-1_15

2020). Furthermore, outpatient mental healthcare, when provided, is often nonspecific and inadequate to address suicidal thoughts and behaviors. Unfortunately, few professionals are trained in evidence-based suicide care (Schmitz et al., 2012), even though promising treatments for suicidal youth exist (see Zullo et al., Chap. 8, this volume).

Pediatric hospitals and academic medical settings are well-positioned to drive innovation by creating comprehensive evidence-driven approaches to reducing suicide risk. Such approaches should incorporate a continuum of upstream prevention programming as well as family-centered acute clinical services. Nationwide Children's Hospital (NCH) is an example of a pediatric hospital with a large Behavioral Health (BH) service line that offers multiple levels of care from prevention through crisis stabilization and inpatient psychiatric care. This chapter will review integration of the Zero Suicide framework into NCH's existing preventable harm reduction quality improvement (QI) initiative to improve clinical care.

Setting the Stage

Zero Suicide is an aspirational goal designed to catalyze transformational change in an organization by providing best practice tools and strategies designed to improve suicide care (www.zerosuicide.edc.org). The Zero Suicide framework is based on three critical factors:

1. Core values that reinforce the belief that suicide can be eliminated by improving service access and quality through continuous quality improvement.
2. Systems management to create a culture that no longer finds suicide to be an acceptable outcome, where aspirational but achievable goals are set to eliminate suicide attempts and deaths and service delivery and supports are organized accordingly.
3. Evidence-based clinical care practices that all staff are trained to provide, delivered consistently across the system of care.

More specifically, Zero Suicide consists of seven elements essential to full implementation:

- Lead system-wide culture change committed to reducing suicides.
- Train a competent, confident, and caring workforce.
- Identify individuals with suicide risk via comprehensive screening and assessment.
- Engage all individuals with suicide risk using a suicide care management plan.
- Treat suicidal thoughts and behaviors using evidence-based treatments.
- Transition individuals through care with warm handoffs and supportive contacts.
- Improve policies and procedures through continuous quality improvement.

Healthcare systems that bundle core components of Zero Suicide show evidence of reduction in patient suicides and suicidal behaviors (Hampton, 2010; Layman et al., 2021; Stapelberg et al., 2021; Turner et al., 2021). Eliminating gaps in suicide safer care requires a comprehensive, system-wide approach, in our case specifically adapted to a pediatric population. The first step for any organization is the completion of the Zero Suicide Organization Self-Study (Zero Suicide, 2021a). This tool helps to identify organizational strengths and gaps and serves as a baseline as well as a needs assessment.

NCH Zero Suicide Organizational Self-Study summary	
Strengths	Gaps
Teams engaged in crisis care had high levels of training	Inconsistent processes for suicide risk screening, evidence-based risk assessment, and safety planning across services
Routine suicide risk assessments administered during diagnostic assessments	Limited input from attempt and loss survivors
Evidence-based suicide risk assessment for programs routinely managing psychiatric crises	Inconsistent suicide-specific training across all programs and disciplines
	Gaps in communication and documentation of prior treatment and safety plans
Suicide-specific treatment programs (e.g., Dialectical Behavior Therapy)	Limited follow-up during transitions in care
	Inconsistent coordination with families and schools

Lead Element of Zero Suicide

As with most organizations that adopt the Zero Suicide framework, successful implementation and incorporation of core values into the culture of NCH's large BH service line required the following:

- Visible support and direction from senior leadership
- Clear expectations for staff, consistent communication, procedures, and workflows demonstrating organizational responsibility for suicide prevention
- Ongoing training and education
- Minimal increase in provider burden including documentation or workload requirements
- Efforts to reduce provider anxiety related to engaging in suicide care and the potential for adverse events

Accordingly, staff across the BH service line were provided an overview of the framework with an overwhelmingly enthusiastic response. The Zero Suicide Workforce Survey (Zero Suicide, 2021b) was then provided to all staff, clinical and nonclinical, with an 80% response rate. The Survey provided a snapshot of staff's self-perception of their competence, comfort, training needs, and perceived skill with regard to providing suicide care which was then used to create a training plan.

Informed by the Workforce Survey results, our approach to training focused on the following:

- Engage clinical leaders (e.g., managers and supervisors) across the service line.
- Review the aims of Zero Suicide and its intent to be both an aspirational goal as well as a specific bundle of interventions.
- Focus initially on the Lead, Train, Identify, and Engage elements, given that some suicide-specific treatments were already part of the continuum of care.
- Standardize skills in screening, assessment, and safety planning in an interactive fashion.
- Develop workflows and process maps flexible enough to tailor for each department.
- Ensure the electronic medical record (EMR) supports decision-making and reduces clinician burden to enhance communication and eliminate duplicate efforts.
- Ensure leaders are able to monitor compliance and provide timely feedback to support staff at different developmental levels.

A key innovation in setting the stage for implementation was the development of an NCH Zero Suicide "Toolkit" as a centralized location in the EMR to house all suicide-specific tools and processes across encounters and levels of care (e.g., automated prompts and workflows for screening, assessment, safety plans, and risk categorization). This information had previously been siloed and difficult to access as patients moved among programs and levels of care, disrupting communication of clinically significant information and leading to inconsistent processes. Workflows were informed by our lived experience champion who provided valuable feedback regarding acceptability to patients while pointing out the frustration of answering the same questions about suicide risk and safety to each new provider in the midst of a crisis. Availability of this toolkit contributed to progress in all seven of the Zero Suicide elements, including "Improve" as it facilitated easy access to process measures. Furthermore, it has been well-received by clinicians who report it does indeed improve access to suicide risk-related information and enhances efficiency.

Train and Engage Elements of Zero Suicide

Training of staff across disciplines and programs laid the foundation for all ongoing Zero Suicide efforts in BH which included a focus on clinician attitudes and biases, supervision strategies, and legal considerations. Clinical competencies addressed were evidence-based screening (Ask Suicide-Screening Questions; Horowitz et al., 2012), risk assessment (Columbia-Suicide Severity Risk Scale; Posner et al., 2011), risk and protective factors, safety planning (Stanley & Brown, 2012), and lethal means safety and risk categorization. Since the initial department-wide series of Zero Suicide trainings, training on suicide care competencies has been incorporated into onboarding processes of all BH teams. An aspect of the Engage element is to create a suicide care management plan based on level of risk. Our risk categorization now clearly identifies those higher-risk youth needing additional services and is visible to all departments across the hospital. A next step is to develop a consistent set of practices across departments for those high-risk youth.

Treat and Transition Elements of Zero Suicide

As reflected in the Self-Study and Workforce Survey summaries, BH services had some programs in which clinicians were highly skilled in treating youth presenting with suicidal thoughts and behaviors and others with low comfort and competence. Guided by the extant literature, NCH had developed a continuum of best practice targeted interventions and suicide-specific treatments. These included a Psychiatric Crisis Department with a strong emphasis on safety planning and lethal means safety, a crisis stabilization unit, inpatient psychiatry units, and intensive outpatient and partial hospitalization programs, in addition to an outpatient Dialectical Behavior Therapy (DBT) program. The Zero Suicide framework helped knit these and other elements into a more cohesive whole and served as a focus for training clinical providers on suicide-specific interventions.

Effectively addressing transitions in care has been difficult, and we have not yet fully implemented a transition care pathway for youth stepping down to a lower level of care. We have attempted to implement warm handoffs, but this can be a challenge in a large hospital system when referrals are made outside the hospital's system of care. On a positive note, NCH has improved care transitions for high acuity youth by adding non-demand caring contacts in the form of validating text messages with images of hope and supportive language sent to adolescents in the year following discharge, regardless of whether they are transitioning within NCH or to an outside agency. We will continue to address the Transitions element by revisiting and formalizing protocols for a transition care pathway supported by review of data to determine linkage, follow-through, and dropout rates.

Improve Element of Zero Suicide

Healthcare organizations implementing Zero Suicide engage in continuous quality improvement (QI) and are able to engage in high-risk work while minimizing serious harm or adverse events. Viewing suicide as a "never event" forces organizations to use best practices, apply continuous QI, and emphasize reducing errors while holding the system accountable, rather than blaming individuals. NCH had an existing commitment to reducing preventable harm via a "Zero Hero" initiative with significant improvements in serious safety events, such as central line catheter infections, using a QI methodology (Miller et al., 2011). Incorporating Zero Suicide was seen as a natural extension of the hospital's QI efforts.

The development of an internal Zero Suicide Toolkit with discrete data elements made it possible to evaluate compliance and set realistic goals for improvement. Initial goals focused on adherence to suicide risk screening with the Ask Suicide-Screening Questions (ASQ) at first visit and every 30 days thereafter, suicide risk assessment with the Columbia-Suicide Severity Risk Scale (C-SSRS), and completion of a safety plan for youth identified as at elevated risk. Within 3 months of implementation, the initial goal of screening >90% of all new patients for suicide risk was met. Focus then shifted to ensuring that all patients with an acute positive screen received a same-day risk assessment and safety plan. After addressing reporting inconsistencies in the EMR, compliance of >93% was quickly established for same-day risk assessment and safety planning. The robustness of a systemic approach to suicide care was demonstrated when screening compliance at first appointment remained consistently in the target range (>90%) after the shift to telehealth at the onset of the pandemic.

A dynamic Zero Suicide dashboard is available to clinical leaders to monitor progress in real time, evaluate the performance of specific programs, and provide feedback to individual providers. In the future, patient care and outcome data will be prioritized, while process measures will continue to be collected to assess fidelity. QI methodology offers the ability to monitor process and treatment outcomes and, using an iterative approach, modify processes to improve patient outcomes (Valleru et al., 2019).

Gaps and Next Steps

The Zero Suicide framework was adopted at NCH in response to a large increase in high acuity patients and a desire to maximize the effectiveness of growing crisis and inpatient services. Over the past 5 years, NCH BH has successfully implemented many best practice elements. What was previously fragmented suicide care is now more intentional, offering staff greater connection to the work and youth and their families more hope for the best possible outcomes. Consistency of implementation and increased staff competence and confidence across the BH workforce effectively means that no matter where youth enter the BH system, they will receive the evidence-based suicide screening and, as appropriate, assessment, safety planning, and intervention. The model has now been adopted by the hospital broadly even outside of BH, and next steps include expansion to other departments starting with those seeing significant numbers of youth with elevated risk, such as primary care. This expansion requires:

- Development of referral pathways that enhance each department's internal capacity to screen and assess for suicide risk, thereby avoiding unnecessary emergent referrals for BH assessments.

- Development of a suicide care pathway wrapping elements of care around patients at highest risk (e.g., immediate follow-up when patients fail to attend an appointment).
- Ongoing monitoring to ensure effective transition of patients among services.
- Ongoing monitoring of communication among providers and departments.

Successful adoption and sustainability of Zero Suicide requires careful planning, supportive infrastructure, and routine review of data aimed at enhancing practice and training. The Zero Suicide model is feasible both in pediatric hospitals and many other healthcare settings, and the release of suicide-specific standards by accrediting bodies has signaled that suicide prevention is a core responsibility of healthcare. However, these standards are still open to interpretation (e.g., frequency of screening) and require further investigation. The use of peer supports or other therapeutic interventions as well as greater specificity regarding risk stratification may help defray the burden on monitoring and environmental controls that currently exists.

Ideally, alternative payment models that support Zero Suicide and suicide-specific care practices would be offered by payers to incentivize this work. It is arguably in the best interests of managed care entities and accountable care organizations to invest in high-quality and effective suicide prevention. Decreased suicide behaviors and improved treatment outcomes should result in patients being supported in less restrictive care settings, decreased healthcare costs, and better experiences of care. Decreased flow to acute care services would, in turn, decrease pressure on the BH system and improve waitlists. This would likely be most effective if providers across communities collaborated to align suicide care practices.

Access to timely care continues to be a challenge, and, as indicated above, even when care is provided, utilization of follow-up referrals tends to be poor. Further investigation into engaging families and high-risk adolescents in treatment is warranted. This includes exploring technology to enhance engagement, increase access, improve lethal means safety and safety planning, and enhance a sense of connectedness. Additionally, using technology helps to increase fidelity to best practices that directly reduce suicide thoughts and behaviors, particularly in the face of a workforce that has variable training and comfort with using suicide-specific interventions.

In summary, Zero Suicide provides a flexible framework for combining best practice suicide care interventions into a comprehensive and systematic approach using real-time data to improve processes and outcomes. There is still a need for more research on the effectiveness of the model and for more systems to share lessons learned as well as how they have managed gaps in care to ease the implementation burden for organizations new to this model. By adopting and striving for the aspirational goal of Zero Suicide and embedding this model's bundle of specific suicide care practices, healthcare systems expressly support their workforce, alter the quality of care provided, and increase patient safety.

References

Asarnow, J. R., Baraff, L. J., Berk, M., Grob, C. S., Devich-Navarro, M., Suddath, R., Piacentini, J. C., Rotheram-Borus, M. J., Cohen, D., & Tang, L. (2011). An emergency department intervention for linking pediatric suicidal patients to follow-up mental health treatment. *Psychiatric Services (Washington, DC), 62*(11), 1303–1309. https://doi.org/10.1176/ps.62.11. pss6211_1303

Burns, C. D., Cortell, R., & Wagner, B. M. (2008). Treatment compliance in adolescents after attempted suicide: A 2-year follow-up study. *Journal of the American Academy of Child and Adolescent Psychiatry, 47*(8), 948–957. https://doi.org/10.1097/CHI.0b013e3181799e84

Chung, D., Hadzi-Pavlovic, D., Wang, M., Swaraj, S., Olfson, M., & Large, M. (2019). Meta-analysis of suicide rates in the first week and the first month after psychiatric hospitalisation. *BMJ Open, 9*(3), e023883. https://doi.org/10.1136/bmjopen-2018-023883

Doupnik, S. K., Rudd, B., Schmutte, T., Worsley, D., Bowden, C., et al. (2020). Association of suicide prevention interventions with subsequent suicide attempts, linkage to follow-up care, and depression symptoms for acute care settings: A systematic review and meta-analysis. *JAMA Psychiatry, 77*(10), 1021–1030. https://doi.org/10.1001/jamapsychiatry.2020.1586

Fontanella, C. A., Warner, L. A., Steelesmith, D. L., Brock, G., Bridge, J. A., & Campo, J. V. (2020). Association of timely outpatient mental health services for youths after psychiatric hospitalization with risk of death by suicide. *JAMA Network Open, 3*(8), e2012887. https://doi.org/10.1001/jamanetworkopen.2020.12887

Goldman-Mellor, S. J., Bhat, H. S., Allen, M. H., & Schoenbaum, M. (2021). Suicide risk among hospitalized versus discharged deliberate self-harm patients: Generalized random forest analysis using a large claims data set. *American Journal of Preventive Medicine*, S0749-3797(21)00516-X. Advance online publication. https://doi.org/10.1016/j.amepre.2021.08.028

Hampton, T. (2010). Depression care effort brings dramatic drop in large HMO population's suicide rate. *JAMA, 303*(19), 1903–1905. https://doi.org/10.1001/jama.2010.595

Horowitz, L. M., Bridge, J. A., Teach, S. J., Ballard, E., Klima, J., Rosenstein, D. L., Wharff, E. A., Ginnis, K., Cannon, E., Joshi, P., & Pao, M. (2012). Ask Suicide-Screening Questions (ASQ): A brief instrument for the pediatric emergency department. *Archives of Pediatrics & Adolescent Medicine, 166*(12), 1170–1176. https://doi.org/10.1001/archpediatrics.2012.1276

Kennard, B., Mayes, T., King, J., Moorehead, A., Wolfe, K., Hughes, J., Castillo, B., Smith, M., Matney, J., Oscarson, B., Stewart, S., Nakonezny, P., Foxwell, A., & Emslie, G. (2019). The development and feasibility outcomes of a youth suicide prevention intensive outpatient program. *The Journal of Adolescent Health, 64*(3), 362–369. https://doi.org/10.1016/j.jadohealth.2018.09.015

Layman, D. M., Kammer, J., Leckman-Westin, E., Hogan, M., Goldstein Grumet, J., Labouliere, C. D., Stanley, B., Carruthers, J., & Finnerty, M. (2021). The relationship between suicidal behaviors and Zero Suicide organizational best practices in outpatient mental health clinics. *Psychiatric Services (Washington, DC), 72*(10), 1118–1125. https://doi.org/10.1176/appi.ps.202000525

Miller, M. R., Niedner, M. F., Huskins, W. C., Colantuoni, E., Yenokyan, G., Moss, M., Rice, T. B., Ridling, D., Campbell, D., Brilli, R. J., & National Association of Children's Hospitals and Related Institutions Pediatric Intensive Care Unit Central Line-Associated Bloodstream Infection Quality Transformation Teams. (2011). Reducing PICU central line-associated bloodstream infections: 3-year results. *Pediatrics, 128*(5), e1077–e1083. https://doi.org/10.1542/peds.2010-3675

National Action Alliance for Suicide Prevention. (2017). *Best practices in care transitions for individuals with suicide risk: Inpatient care to outpatient care.* https://www.samhsa.gov/sites/default/files/suicide-risk-practices-in-care-transitions-11192019.pdf

Plemmons, G., Hall, M., Doupnik, S., Gay, J., Brown, C., Browning, W., Casey, R., Freundlich, K., Johnson, D. P., Lind, C., Rehm, K., Thomas, S., & Williams, D. (2018). Hospitalization for suicide ideation or attempt: 2008-2015. *Pediatrics, 141*(6), e20172426. https://doi.org/10.1542/peds.2017-2426

Posner, K., Brown, G. K., Stanley, B., Brent, D. A., Yershova, K. V., Oquendo, M. A., Currier, G. W., Melvin, G. A., Greenhill, L., Shen, S., & Mann, J. J. (2011). The Columbia-Suicide Severity Rating Scale: Initial validity and internal consistency findings from three multisite studies with adolescents and adults. *The American Journal of Psychiatry, 168*(12), 1266–1277. https://doi.org/10.1176/appi.ajp.2011.10111704

Schmitz, W. M., Jr., Allen, M. H., Feldman, B. N., Gutin, N. J., Jahn, D. R., Kleespies, P. M., Quinnett, P., & Simpson, S. (2012). Preventing suicide through improved training in suicide risk assessment and care: An American association of suicidology task force report addressing serious gaps in U.S. mental health training. *Suicide & Life-Threatening Behavior, 42*(3), 292–304. https://doi.org/10.1111/j.1943-278X.2012.00090.x

Spirito, A., Simon, V., Cancilliere, M. K., Stein, R., Norcott, C., Loranger, K., & Prinstein, M. J. (2011). Outpatient psychotherapy practice with adolescents following psychiatric hospitalization for suicide ideation or a suicide attempt. *Clinical Child Psychology and Psychiatry, 16*(1), 53–64. https://doi.org/10.1177/1359104509352893

Stanley, B., & Brown, G. K. (2012). Safety planning intervention: A brief intervention to mitigate suicide risk. *Cognitive and Behavioral Practice, 19*(2), 256–264. https://doi.org/10.1016/j.cbpra.2011.01.001

Stapelberg, N., Sveticic, J., Hughes, I., Almeida-Crasto, A., Gaee-Atefi, T., Gill, N., Grice, D., Krishnaiah, R., Lindsay, L., Patist, C., Engelen, H. V., Walker, S., Welch, M., Woerwag-Mehta, S., & Turner, K. (2021). Efficacy of the Zero Suicide framework in reducing recurrent suicide attempts: Cross-sectional and time-to-recurrent-event analyses. *The British Journal of Psychiatry: the Journal of Mental Science, 219*(2), 427–436. https://doi.org/10.1192/bjp.2020.190

Turner, K., Sveticic, J., Almeida-Crasto, A., Gaee-Atefi, T., Green, V., Grice, D., Kelly, P., Krishnaiah, R., Lindsay, L., Mayahle, B., Patist, C., Van Engelen, H., Walker, S., Welch, M., Woerwag-Mehta, S., & Stapelberg, N. J. (2021). Implementing a systems approach to suicide prevention in a mental health service using the Zero Suicide Framework. *The Australian and New Zealand Journal of Psychiatry, 55*(3), 241–253. https://doi.org/10.1177/0004867420971698

Valleru, J., Krishna, R., & Fristad, M. A. (2019). Systemic approach to successful quality improvement in behavioral health. *Evidence-Based Practice in Child and Adolescent Mental Health, 4*(4), 344–356. https://doi.org/10.1080/23794925.2019.1685417

Zero Suicide. (2021a). Zero Suicide Organizational Self-Study. *Education Development Center.* https://zerosuicide.edc.org/resources/key-resources/organizational-self-study

Zero Suicide. (2021b). Zero Suicide Workforce Survey. *Education Development Center.* https://go.edc.org/ZSWorkforceSurvey

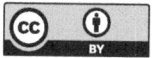

Chapter 16
Suicide Prevention for American Indian and Alaska Native Youth: Lessons Learned and Implications for Underserved Communities

Mary F. Cwik, Teresa Brockie, Sarah M. Edwards, Holly C. Wilcox, and John V. Campo

Suicide is a serious and universal public health challenge, yet significant disparities have been observed in suicide and attempt rates across a variety of cultural, racial, and ethnic subgroups. A better understanding of differences among cultural, racial, and ethnic subgroups with regard to suicide and suicidal behavior has the potential to inform suicide prevention efforts, not only within these specific subgroups but in general populations as well. This chapter will focus on the American Indian and Alaska Native (AI/AN) population as illustrative of several best practices and lessons learned with implications for other underserved communities, as well as calls to action for the field more broadly.

M. F. Cwik (✉) · H. C. Wilcox
Johns Hopkins Bloomberg School of Public Health, Baltimore, MD, USA

Johns Hopkins School of Medicine, Baltimore, MD, USA
e-mail: mcwik1@jhu.edu; hwilcox1@jhmi.edu

T. Brockie
Johns Hopkins School of Nursing, Baltimore, MD, USA
e-mail: tbrocki1@jhu.edu

S. M. Edwards
University of Maryland School of Medicine, Baltimore, MD, USA
e-mail: sedwards@som.umaryland.edu

J. V. Campo
Johns Hopkins School of Medicine, Baltimore, MD, USA
e-mail: jcampo3@jhmi.edu

© The Author(s) 2022
J. P. Ackerman, L. M. Horowitz (eds.), *Youth Suicide Prevention and Intervention*, SpringerBriefs in Psychology,
https://doi.org/10.1007/978-3-031-06127-1_16

Epidemiology of Suicide in AI/AN Communities

AI/AN communities have some of the highest suicide rates among youth (see Ruch and Bridge, Chap. 1, this volume), although there is considerable heterogeneity in rates across AI/AN communities. Suicide was the leading cause of death in 10–14-year-old AI/AN males in the United States in 2019. Notably, the suicide rate among AI/AN males has increased from 17.3 per 100,000 in 2001 to 20.3 per 100,000 in 2019 and 3.9 per 100,000 to 6.9 per 100,000 in AI/AN females—a 77% increase for females vs. a 17% increase for males. Suicide rates in all male race/ethnicity groups increase sharply to age 20–24, with AI/AN male suicide rates far surpassing those of all other groups at this age bracket. Comparing across all male racial/ethnic groups, AI/AN males have the highest suicide rate until age 40–44.

Despite these significant disparities in suicide rates, suicide prevention in underserved populations has been limited by critical gaps in research, training, and program implementation. Moreover, these underserved populations, such as AI/AN communities, are often not represented in national epidemiological studies in a meaningful way. This underrepresentation contributes to invisibility. Native Americans, for example, are often put in an "other" category or lumped together with other racial/ethnic groups with small numbers in the sample. Consequently, large-scale data describing suicide in a Native context are relatively lacking, making it difficult to appropriately direct funding and to further make an argument to purposively include Natives and other underrepresented minorities in large-scale clinical trials. As a result, there appears to be a lack of "evidence-based" interventions for underserved communities, even though AI/AN populations have championed several important innovations that have often been ignored by the larger suicide prevention field, including being early advocates for strengths-based and community-based approaches, developing frugal interventions, harnessing the power of early identification in community settings, and emphasizing culture and spirituality as part of holistic approaches.

Best Practices in Underserved Communities

Strengths- and Community-Based Approaches

A shift from a deficits-based approach to suicide prevention, which focuses on individual-level risk factors and psychopathology, to a strengths-based approach is underway in underserved communities and timely for the rest of the field (Tingey et al., 2016; Yuan et al., 2015). While deficits-based approaches can guide individual risk mitigation efforts, they also have the potential to inadvertently contribute to individual and group stigmatization and overemphasize problems in communities. Deficit models are not always effective either; decades of suicide prevention work and federal government-funded programs applying deficit models have not reduced the high prevalence of suicide in Indian country. Utilizing a deficits-based approach might even prove harmful to marginalized communities and hinder their ability to adequately address suicide. Conversely, strengths-based approaches highlight community and cultural protective factors and involve community members to promote well-being and positive health outcomes. For example, one strengths-based approach for addressing substance use and suicide utilizes a positive youth development framework to provide an entrepreneurship education intervention for White Mountain Apache youth (Tingey et al., 2016). Additionally, the Sources of Strength program employs effective public health messaging and stories of personal resilience in managing emotions for upstream suicide prevention (Thiha et al., 2016). The field of suicide prevention, in general, can learn from the community-based participatory research process that is the foundation for many strengths-based approaches, which has building trust as the foundation of successful research, regardless of whether the researchers are considered "insiders" or "outsiders" (Wallerstein & Duran, 2010).

Frugal Interventions

The scarcity of mental health services and providers has required underserved communities to develop "frugal innovations." Frugal innovations in mental or public health sectors can be thought of as interventions that do more with less, capable of reaching the many. There are few sustained programs that address community mental health needs, especially those that focus on suicide prevention. Programs tend not to detail specific risk and protective factors identified in remote, resource-poor settings. The frugal intervention development process—*whereby, in limited resources settings, creativity and imagination have better opportunities to develop*—goes beyond addressing limitations based upon external resource constraints. Such a model enhances an understanding of self-reliant processes and internal resources that are often overlooked. The suicide prevention field needs to develop new solutions in resource-challenged settings rather than relying on untested adaptations often developed far away in well-resourced communities (Lorini, 2016). One type of frugal intervention model that Native and other underserved communities support is a brief intervention delivered by community health workers. For example, a pilot study evaluated the potential effectiveness of a specific brief intervention, New Hope, with findings indicating reductions in negative thinking, depression, and suicidal thoughts among youth with a history of suicide attempt (Cwik et al. 2016a).

Early Identification in Community Settings

Suicide surveillance is often viewed as an important way to identify individuals at risk for suicide. Community-based identification is especially important in under-served communities relative to hospital- and clinic-based approaches to case identi-fication since there are many barriers to vulnerable youth accessing care. The White Mountain Apache Tribe has developed an innovative and effective system that man-dates any person who lives or works on the reservation to report any suicide-related incident (ideation, attempt, and death) to a central task force called Celebrating Life (CL). After a report is made, a CL staff member follows up in person to gather more information on risk and protective factors, enable a warm handoff to services, and provide case management. This is both an innovative and culturally acceptable way of delivering services to those most at risk for suicide. This system gives the Tribe accurate, timely, and thorough data on suicide in their community, allowing them to target suicide prevention efforts. Over time, surveillance has raised community awareness, identified many individuals at risk for suicide, and increased the percent-age of those getting referrals for treatment. The initial surveillance data resulted in a comprehensive program that included universal, selected, and indicated suicide prevention activities; this multitiered approach was associated with a significant reduction in suicide attempts and deaths (Cwik et al., 2016b).

Holistic Approaches

Approaches that incorporate culture and/or spirituality have potential to contribute to both prevention and treatment, particularly in AI/AN communities. Elders from the White Mountain Apache Reservation, for example, have focused on the impor-tance of their culture and language to prevent suicide, developing a standardized curriculum that they have been teaching in schools since 2014 (Cwik et al., 2019). The Elders believe that language provides youth with a solid sense of self, tribal identity, and connection to the community, all of which serve as protective factors. Respect is a core value addressed across all the lessons, and the monthly content corresponds with what is traditionally taught at that time of year with a different theme for each lesson/month. Youth learn Apache words, stories, and seasonal responsibilities related to that month's theme. Students reported high program satis-faction and displayed knowledge of their culture and language on written assess-ments after participating (Cwik et al., 2019). Finally, many underserved communities are already implementing programs which they believe to be effective in their set-tings, and do not feel a need for evidence in the form of a randomized clinical trial. As a larger scientific field, we often do not know about community perceptions about the success of these local efforts or dismiss them, with potentially negative consequences for developing and advancing evidence-based suicide prevention efforts in underserved communities. Some traditional suicide prevention approaches, terminology, and interventions are not viewed as acceptable or culturally congruent. For instance, "gatekeeper" programs have been implemented in tribal communities, often with adaptations, but this terminology has been replaced with "caretaker" to avoid negative conations associated with the idea that "gatekeepers" might exclude some individuals. Examples of culturally congruent, strength-based programs can be found in the Culture Forward guide (https://caih.jhu.edu/programs/cultureforward) and include the Healing of the Canoe project, the Qungasvik Toolbox, the Yappali Project and Culture Camps, and Native H.O.P.E. (Helping Our People Endure).

Call to Action

There are two overarching calls to action for what suicide prevention research, policy, and practice can learn from underserved communities. First and most importantly, we need to diversify the suicide prevention field, both in terms of who is being included in our study populations and who is conducting the research. It is imperative to include underserved communities in research so that we have better data (and interventions) moving forward. Furthermore, developing more independent investigators and funded researchers from underserved communities has potential to advance suicide prevention efforts, not just in vulnerable populations but in general. Researchers and clinicians from the same racial/ethnic group are more likely to be sensitive to, understand, and appreciate the cultural norms and values, past and current traumas, and language issues relevant to the study of suicide risk and protective factors and preventive interventions. From a clinical perspective, training more providers from underserved communities has potential to be an important contribution to the continuum of care relevant to suicide prevention efforts. In addition, having a provider from the same racial/ethnic group can provide comfort and security for some individuals at risk for suicide, and may feel less stigmatizing, enhancing the likelihood that individuals will reach out for help and stay in treatment. Additionally, providers from other communities need more training on the process and content specific to addressing suicide in underserved communities. Many providers lack suicide prevention training generally, but the nuances of working with underserved communities are rarely addressed in training programs. Policies with funding and specific programs attached to it are urgently needed to focus on increasing the diversity of the workforce and mandating these types of trainings at the federal, state, and institutional level.

Second, suicide prevention programs need to be developed with sustainability in mind, which is critically important in underserved communities. Although seeking community buy-in would intuitively seem to be an important first step in suicide prevention, policy makers, funders, and researchers have often failed to put this principle into action. We need to begin with an approach that includes listening to the community with a sense of openness and curiosity, tailoring prevention efforts to the community at risk instead of fitting the community to an established program. It is also vital to understand the effort, training, and supervision required for local communities to enact best practices. Implementing a "train the trainer" approach is often more productive than relying exclusively on "outsiders"; there is wisdom in being open to community health worker delivery models for practical and cultural reasons. Finally, policy makers, researchers, and individuals in clinical leadership roles need to identify sustainable funding streams and innovative service delivery models (O'Keefe et al., 2021)—as prevention programs may be particularly challenging to deliver with fidelity in underserved communities, who may feel a sense of abandonment when initial grant funding comes to an end.

Conclusions

The study of underserved communities has potential to contribute to suicide prevention efforts for both underserved communities and the general population. Researchers, policy makers, and clinicians can no longer afford to ignore what is happening in underserved communities. Focused research can inform the efforts of health policy experts and lawmakers to mitigate disparities and improve access to high-quality, evidence-based mental health and substance use services for all. Priority research targets should include ensuring that Native American and other racial/ethnic groups are represented in large-scale or national epidemiological studies in a meaningful way; understanding root causes of suicide beyond individual-level factors (e.g., past and current traumas, socioeconomic conditions); and innovative models of prevention and intervention focused on holistic well-being. Our shared humanity makes suicide a problem that transcends specific cultural, ethnic, or racial groups; however, it is also true that cultural, ethnic, and racial differences can be associated with differences in rates of suicide and suicidal behaviors, suggesting the need for both universal and targeted approaches to suicide prevention in subpopulations of individuals at risk, particularly in the underserved. A better understanding of suicide in underserved communities has potential to improve the quality and effectiveness of interventions in those communities, inform the adaptation of successful suicide prevention strategies to specific subpopulations, motivate the creation of new programs, and contribute to our understanding of suicide and suicide prevention in general.

References

Cwik, M. F., Tingey, L., Lee, A., Suttle, R., Lake, K., Walkup, J. T., & Barlow, A. (2016a). Development and piloting of a brief intervention for suicidal American Indian adolescents. *American Indian and Alaska Native Mental Health Research, 23*, 105–124. https://doi-org.proxy1.library.jhu.edu/10.5820/aian.2301.2016.105

Cwik, M. F., Tingey, L., Maschino, A., Goklish, N., Larzelere-Hinton, F., Walkup, J., & Barlow, A. (2016b). Decreases in suicide deaths and attempts linked to the white mountain apache suicide surveillance and prevention system, 2001–2012. *American Journal of Public Health, 106*(12), 2183–2189. https://doi-org.proxy1.library.jhu.edu/10.2105/AJPH.2016.303453

Cwik, M. F., Goklish, N., Masten, K., Lee, A., Suttle, R., Alchesay, M., O'Keefe, V., & Barlow, A. (2019). "Let our Apache Heritage and culture live on forever and teach the young ones": Development of The elders' resilience curriculum, an upstream suicide prevention approach for American Indian Youth. *American Journal of Community Psychology, 64*(1-2), 137–145. https://doi-org.proxy1.library.jhu.edu/10.1002/ajcp.12351

Lorini, M. R. (2016). *Collective creative processes in underserved contexts: Lessons of grassroots frugal social innovations.* Paper presented at 8th annual SIG GlobDev conference. http://aisel.aisnet.org/globdev2016/2

O'Keefe, V. M., Cwik, M. F., Haroz, E. E., & Barlow, A. (2021). Increasing culturally responsive care and mental health equity with indigenous community mental health workers. *Psychological Services, 18*(1), 84–92. https://doi-org.proxy1.library.jhu.edu/10.1037/ser0000358.

Thiha, P., Pisani, A. R., Gurditta, K., Cherry, E., Peterson, D. R., Kautz, H., & Wyman, P. A. (2016). Efficacy of web-based collection of strength-based testimonials for text message extension of youth suicide prevention program: Randomized controlled experiment. *JMIR Public Health and Surveillance, 2*(2), e164. https://doi-org.proxy1.library.jhu.edu/10.2196/publichealth.6207.

Tingey, L., Larzelere-Hinton, F., Goklish, N., Ingalls, A., Craft, T., Sprengeler, F., McGuire, C., & Barlow, A. (2016). Entrepreneurship education: A strength-based approach to substance use and suicide prevention for American Indian adolescents. *American Indian and Alaska Native Mental Health Research, 23*(3), 248–270. https://doi-org.proxy1.library.jhu.edu/10.5820/aian.2303.2016.248

Wallerstein, N., & Duran, B. (2010). Community-based participatory research contributions to intervention research: The intersection of science and practice to improve health equity. *American Journal of Public Health, 100*(Suppl 1), S40–S46. https://doi.org/10.2105/AJPH.2009.184036

Yuan, N. P., Belcourt-Dittloff, A., Schultz, K., Packard, G., & Duran, B. M. (2015). Research agenda for violence against American Indian and Alaska Native women: Toward the development of strength-based and resilience interventions. *Psychology of Violence, 5*(4), 367–373. https://doi.org/10.1037/a0038507

Chapter 17
Overcoming Barriers to Effective Suicide Prevention in Rural Communities

Kurt D. Michael and Ujjwal Ramtekkar

Rising suicide rates, the opioid crisis, and persisting healthcare disparities have collectively created a perfect storm of factors associated with higher rates of premature death in rural communities. Unfortunately, rural communities often experience disproportionate suicide rates compared to urban settings (Fontanella et al., 2015). Moreover, the capacity of the healthcare systems in most rural communities has been in steady decline for years. This capacity problem is due, in part, to the closing of rural hospitals and clinics and workforce shortages in remote regions (Thomas et al., 2012). These workforce and clinic shortages are exacerbated by other barriers, including economic disparities (e.g., lack of insurance), geographic remoteness, inadequate transportation, and a lack of sufficient infrastructure for telehealth solutions.

Acceptability of mental health services or lack thereof also acts as a barrier to effective suicide prevention in rural communities. It is not an uncommon perception in small communities that disclosing personal health information to a medical or mental health professional is unnecessary, unhelpful, or a sign of being disloyal to the family (Owens et al., 2013). Similarly, individuals from rural areas have also reported that receiving conventional mental health care signals weakness or indicates that one has spiritual flaws (Curtin et al., 2017).

Easy access to lethal means, primarily firearms and dangerous medications, also makes it difficult to prevent suicide in rural regions. Between 1999 and 2019, the leading mechanism of suicide for youth aged 10–19 living in the least populous

K. D. Michael (✉)
Appalachian State University, Boone, NC, USA
e-mail: michaelkd@appstate.edu

U. Ramtekkar
University of Missouri School of Medicine, Columbia, MO, USA

Teladoc Health Inc., Jefferson City, MO, USA
e-mail: ramtekkaru@health.missouri.edu

© The Author(s) 2022
J. P. Ackerman, L. M. Horowitz (eds.), *Youth Suicide Prevention
and Intervention*, SpringerBriefs in Psychology,
https://doi.org/10.1007/978-3-031-06127-1_17

(rural) areas of the United States was firearms (56%), whereas firearm suicides in this age group overall was lower (46%; CDC WONDER, 2021). Ready access to prescription opioids in rural Appalachia has been well-documented (Meit et al., 2017), and increased access to any prescription or over-the-counter medication in a crisis can lead to increased suicide attempts. The barriers described here, though certainly not exhaustive, are major impediments to the planning and implementation of effective youth suicide prevention strategies in rural settings. Despite these barriers, school mental health partnerships and telehealth models have shown promise in addressing them. These two innovations will be discussed in detail with an emphasis on how they can lead to effective suicide prevention implementation in rural communities.

School Mental Health Innovations for Suicide Prevention

The potential suicide of a student is a serious concern for many K–12 educators and administrators. Results from the 2019 Youth Risk Behavior Survey indicate that 18.8% of teens seriously considered suicide, 8.9% reported at least one suicide attempt, and 2.5% said that they made an attempt that required medical treatment during the previous 12 months (Ivey-Stephenson et al., 2020). As discussed elsewhere in this volume, the epidemiological trends of youth depression, hopelessness, suicidal thoughts, and suicide deaths are sobering (see Bridge et al., this volume). Identifying and treating youth suicidal thoughts and behaviors as early as possible is optimal; however, reaching youth who are at risk presents logistical and practical challenges in rural communities. This makes serving youth where they spend the majority of their time, in the school context, particularly important. However, most schools are already overburdened, and therefore suicide prevention efforts in schools will only succeed if community partners are also committed to reducing existing burdens placed on teachers, counselors, social workers, and administrators, which includes minimizing the negative impact on instruction time.

Assessment, Support, and Counseling (ASC) Centers

In rural western North Carolina, a model of early detection, service provision, and proactive suicide prevention has been implemented, sustained, and evaluated in several rural K–12 districts. The partnerships, called Assessment, Support, and Counseling (ASC) Centers, serve 10–30% of enrolled students annually. These centers represent a creative approach to improving access and acceptability for mental health and suicide prevention services (Albright et al., 2013). ASC Centers are staffed by licensed mental health professionals and graduate trainees under supervision by faculty from various human service disciplines, including clinical psychology, social work, and marriage and family therapy. Thus, in addition to serving youth in the context where they spend the majority of their time during the day, ASC Centers have the capacity and expertise to assist schools and communities to address the problem of suicide directly.

A typical course of treatment for students who access these services includes 10–14 sessions of individualized cognitive behavioral therapy (CBT) over about 2–3 months. Each session lasts about 40 min to minimize the loss of instruction time. ASC Center services have been shown to be effective for the majority of youth receiving them (Albright et al., 2013; Kirk et al., 2019), including significant symptom reduction following treatment of mood disorders (Michael et al., 2016). ASC treatment has also been associated with improved academic outcomes (e.g., better attendance, fewer discipline referrals). Moreover, a signature feature of the ASC Center is the development and implementation of effective and sustainable practices to assess, treat, and manage youth who present with suicidal crises in the context of under-resourced rural school districts. Evidence-based assessments and interventions including CBT, Counseling on Access to Lethal Means (CALM), safe storage of firearms and dangerous medications, the Collaborative Assessment and Management of Suicidality (CAMS), and the use of tangible safety plans as part of CALM and CAMS have been implemented successfully under the auspices of the ASC Model (Capps et al., 2019; Jobes et al., 2019; Kirk et al., 2019).

Telehealth Innovations for Suicide Prevention

In addition to integrated school mental health models, technology represents a way to overcome traditional barriers in rural communities. Over the past few decades, there have been significant strides in deploying tele-behavioral health (TBH) solutions for mental health issues with outcomes that are often equivalent to traditional in-person care. Most youth are well versed in using digital platforms for schoolwork, creative expression, and social engagement, making them "digital natives" who readily accept and adopt evolving technologies (Nesi, 2020). Using digital platforms to deliver mental health care is therefore a feasible and acceptable method of service provision for most youth. Despite the upside of such approaches and the emerging evidence base, there have been barriers in adopting TBH. These include inflexibility of regulating bodies, interstate variability in legal requirements for privacy and security, licensure guidelines that restrict reimbursement, insurance coverage limitations, and an inadequately trained TBH workforce. A silver lining of the COVID-19 pandemic is that the process of pivoting to remote practice methods has accelerated dramatically and readiness to adopt these strategies has likely increased.

One of the persisting barriers to TBH is inconsistent access to broadband connectivity and high-speed data-enabled phone services in rural communities. Even when there is adequate connectivity, socio-economic disparities that are prominent in rural communities have exacerbated existing access barriers. It can be challenging for families to afford to purchase the necessary equipment for TBH, such as smart phones or camera-equipped laptops (Benda et al., 2020). Overcoming access and acceptability barriers to suicide prevention in rural communities ideally involves the merger of the two primary innovations highlighted in this chapter, that is, coupling TBH and school mental health partnerships while seeking funding from local companies and mental health boards as well as small grants from school boards. Such funding can help to offset costs of technological supports (e.g., remote hot spots) and the clinical labor necessary to implement effective suicide prevention programming (Michael, 2020).

School-Based Tele-Behavioral Health (TBH)

School-based health centers and K–12 partnerships have been among the most important drivers of TBH for both medical and behavioral health needs of students. These innovations are now increasingly common in rural and urban schools given the recognition that educational settings are often the hub of the community and that embedding services in schools improves access and acceptability to healthcare treatment, including the normalization of help-seeking (Stephan et al., 2016). The use of TBH in tandem with CAMS in K–12 schools has been especially important during the pandemic leveraging virtual instruction as a way to increase access and reduce negative health outcomes and interruptions to student learning (Jobes et al., 2020). Providing TBH in schools is a practical method of offering a full continuum of student mental health services ranging from building-wide universal mental health promotion to classroom-based education on suicide prevention, tertiary-level crisis intervention, outpatient treatment, and referral. There have been several demonstrably feasible school-based TBH programs established over the past decade (Stephan et al., 2016), and these include an array of services including traditional ambulatory care, case coordination, suicide risk assessment, triage, and crisis management for students. Some models such as COPE (Community Outreach in Pediatrics/Psychiatry and Education) program for elementary schools include stepped care approach of inter-professional consultation with pediatrician in the school-based health clinic followed by telehealth-based psychiatric evaluation (McLennan et al., 2008), whereas other programs are designed for delivering direct therapy independently (Nelson & Patton, 2016) or through the existing network of school health clinics (North, 2020). The available literature provides insights on design and implementation of these programs, but evaluation of longitudinal effectiveness is still needed.

Project ECHO

Project ECHO (Extension for Community Healthcare Outcomes) is an established TBH model that has the potential to bridge some of the prominent barriers to suicide prevention services in rural communities, including K–12 schools. Project ECHO is considered to be a national model for rural health care overall. It is a "hub and spoke" model of telehealth that connects an interdisciplinary hub of experts to spokes of remotely located constituents. It builds local capacity by teaching best practices via case-based learning, video technology, and program evaluation (Zhou et al., 2016).

The composition of the subject matter experts (hub) and the trainings are tailored to meet the needs of the communities or schools (spokes). The interdisciplinary subject matter experts can include psychiatrists, psychologists, social workers, counselors, family advocates, and administrators. Similarly, the "spokes" could be either specific provider groups (e.g., school social workers, counselors) or various constituents such as teachers, nurses, and administrators depending on the needs of the school. The ECHO sessions are then conducted at a regular frequency for the duration of 3–6 months with the same cohort of learners but should be flexible based on school schedules. The didactic content and the case discussions can be tailored to provide the cohorts with high quality, individually tailored training in the prevention, assessment, case conceptualization, intervention, and management of youth at risk for self-harm and suicide. It also overcomes the need to travel long distances to academic medical centers, regional meetings, or national conferences.

Conclusions and Policy Recommendations

There are a number of well-documented barriers when planning and implementing suicide prevention strategies in rural communities. However, school mental health partnerships and TBH innovations represent two approaches that have shown considerable promise in overcoming known impediments to service provision and the prevention of youth suicide in remote settings. Clinicians, program developers, educators, policymakers, and researchers are encouraged to consider four specific recommendations when attempting to address these aforementioned barriers.

First, those interested in school mental health partnerships and telehealth solutions for suicide prevention in rural communities are strongly encouraged to include evidence-based, suicide-specific therapeutic assessments and management paradigms, such as CAMS, as a key feature of their programming. Second, developers and implementers should focus on promoting means reduction principles, including the consistent use of safety plans in their work with patients and families. Some states (e.g., North Carolina) have applied for and received federal funding through the CDC to provide and sustain CALM trainings for mental health clinicians and organizations statewide. Similarly, community agencies, K–12 schools, and health departments should consider partnering with local gun shops and community members invested in firearm safety, proper medication disposal, and safe storage programs to reduce suicide death overall (see Harvard's Means Matter website for a review: https://www.hsph.harvard.edu/means-matter/gun-shop-project/). Third, K–12 partners in rural communities should consider the specific guidance by Schorr et al. (2017) and implement already established evidence-based suicide prevention programs in rural schools. The two programs that have the strongest evidence are Signs of Suicide (SOS; Aseltine et al., 2007) and Lifelines: A Comprehensive Suicide Awareness and Responsiveness Program for Teens (Underwood & Kalafat, 2009). Schorr et al. (2017) also provide a considerable amount of guidance for implementing effective suicide prevention programs across the multitiered systems of support (MTSS) framework in the context of rural schools. Lastly, those interested in scaling up TBH solutions should apply for federal grants like the Distance Learning and Telemedicine (DLT) Program offered by US Department of Agriculture and consider implementing a suicide-specific program such as CAMS, especially in light of recent innovations developed during the COVID-19 pandemic (e.g., Jobes et al., 2020). Investments in rural communities will help curb youth suicide rates in settings, but understanding how to navigate their specific barriers and opportunities is critical.

References

Albright, A., Michael, K. D., Massey, C. S., Sale, R., Kirk, A., & Egan, T. E. (2013). An evaluation of an interdisciplinary rural school mental health program in Appalachia. *Advances in School Mental Health Promotion, 6*, 189–202.

Aseltine, R. H., Jr., James, A., Schilling, E. A., & Glanovsky, J. (2007). Evaluating the SOS suicide prevention program: A replication and extension. *BMC Public Health, 7*, 161. https://doi.org/10.1186/1471-2458-7-161

Benda, N. C., Veinot, T. C., Sieck, C. J., & Ancker, J. S. (2020). Broadband internet access is a social determinant of health! *American Journal of Public Health, 110*(8), 1123–1125. https://doi.org/10.2105/AJPH.2020.305784

Capps, R. E., Michael, K. D., & Jameson, J. P. (2019). Lethal means and adolescent suicide risk: An expansion of the PEACE Protocol. *Journal of Rural Mental Health, 43*(1), 3–16. http://dx.doi.org/10.1037/rmh0000108

Centers for Disease Control and Prevention. (2021). *CDC WONDER.* Retrieved from https://wonder.cdc.gov on February 1, 2021.

Curtin, L., Massey, C., & Keefe, S. E. (2017). Intergenerational and familial influences on mental illness in rural settings and their relevance for school mental health. In K. Michael & J. Jameson (Eds.), *Handbook of rural school mental health.* Springer. https://doi.org/10.1007/978-3-319-64735-7_18

Fontanella, C. A., Hiance-Steelesmith, D. L., Phillips, G. S., Bridge, J. A., Lester, N., Sweeney, H. A., & Campo, J. V. (2015). Widening ruralurban disparities in youth suicides, United States, 1996–2010. *Journal of the American Medical Association Pediatrics, 169*, 466–473. https://dx.doi.org/10.1001/jamapediatrics.2014.3561

Ivey-Stephenson, A. Z., Demissie, Z., Crosby, A. E., Stone, D. M., Gaylor, E., Wilkins, N., Lowry, R., & Brown, M. (2020). Suicidal ideation and behaviors among high school students – Youth Risk Behavior Survey, United States, 2019. *Morbidity and Mortality Weekly Report, 69*(Suppl-1), 47–55.

Jobes, D. A., Vergara, G. A., Lanzillo, E. C., & Ridge-Anderson, A. (2019). The potential use of CAMS for suicidal youth: Building on epidemiology and clinical interventions. *Children's Health Care, 48*(4), 444–468. https://doi.org/10.1080/02739615.2019.1630279

Jobes, D. A., Crumlish, J. A., & Evans, A. D. (2020). The COVID-19 pandemic and treating suicidal risk: The telepsychotherapy use of CAMS. *Journal of Psychotherapy Integration, 30*(2), 226–237. https://doi.org/10.1037/int0000208

Kirk, A., Michael, K., Bergman, S., Schorr, M., & Jameson, J. P. (2019). Dose response effects of cognitive-behavioral therapy in a school mental health program. *Cognitive Behaviour Therapy, 48*(6), 497–516. https://doi.org/10.1080/16506073.2018.1550527

McLennan, J. D., Reckord, M., & Clarke, M. (2008). A mental health outreach program for elementary schools. *Journal of the Canadian Academy of Child and Adolescent Psychiatry, 17*(3), 122–130.

Meit, M., Hefferman, M., Tanenbaum, E., & Hoffmann, T. (2017). *Final report: Appalachian diseases of despair.* Walsh Center for Rural Health Analysis, NORC at the University of Chicago. https://www.arc.gov/wp-content/uploads/2020/06/AppalachianDiseasesofDespairAugust2017.pdf

Michael, K. D. (2020). Youth mental health in North Carolina: Creative innovations in challenging times. *North Carolina Medical Journal, 81*(2), 101–105. https://doi.org/10.18043/ncm.81.2.101

Michael, K. D., George, M. W., Splett, J. W., Jameson, J. P., Sale, R., Albright Bode, A., Iachini, A. L., Taylor, L. K., & Weist, M. D. (2016). Preliminary outcomes of a multi-site, school-based modular intervention for adolescents experiencing mood difficulties. *Journal of Child and Family Studies, 25*(6), 1903–1915.

Nelson, E. L., & Patton, S. (2016). Using videoconferencing to deliver individual therapy and pediatric psychology interventions with children and adolescents. *Journal of Child and Adolescent Psychopharmacology, 26*(3), 212–220. https://doi.org/10.1089/cap.2015.0021

Nesi, J. (2020). The impact of social media on youth mental health. *North Carolina Medical Journal, 81*(2), 116–121. https://doi.org/10.18043/ncm.81.2.116

North, S. (2020). Addressing students' mental health needs via telehealth. *North Carolina Medical Journal, 81*(2), 112–113. https://doi.org/10.18043/ncm.81.2.112

Owens, J. S., Watabe, Y., & Michael, K. D. (2013). Culturally responsive school mental health in rural communities. In C. Clauss-Ehlers, Z. Serpell, & M. Weist (Eds.), *Handbook of culturally responsive school mental health.* Springer. https://doi.org/10.1007/978-1-4614-4948-5_3

Schorr, M., Van Sant, W., & Jameson, J. P. (2017). Preventing suicide among students in rural schools. In K. Michael & J. Jameson (Eds.), *Handbook of rural school mental health.* Springer. https://doi.org/10.1007/978-3-319-64735-7_9

Stephan, S., Lever, N., Bernstein, L., Edwards, S., & Pruitt, D. (2016). Telemental health in schools. *Journal of Child and Adolescent Psychopharmacology, 26*(3), 266–272. https://doi.org/10.1089/cap.2015.0019

Thomas, D., Macdowell, M., & Glasser, M. (2012). Rural mental health workforce needs assessment – A national survey. *Rural and Remote Health, 12,* 2176.

Underwood, M., & Kalafat, J. (2009). *Lifelines: A suicide prevention program.* Hazelden.

Zhou, C., Crawford, A., Serhal, E., Kurdyak, P., & Sockalingam, S. (2016). The impact of Project ECHO on participant and patient outcomes: A systematic review. *Academic Medicine, 91*(10), 1439–1461. https://doi.org/10.1097/ACM.0000000000001328

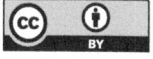

Chapter 18
Disclosure of Youth Suicidality: Views from Lived Experience

Rowan Willis-Powell, Amanda Fox, and Julie Cerel

Living through a suicide attempt gives one a critical perspective that has not been consistently incorporated into treatment and suicide prevention approaches. The engagement of people who are willing to draw from their own experiences of being impacted by suicidal thoughts or behaviors (STB) to advocate for others with similar experiences is foundational to effective suicide prevention. Individuals who identify as suicide attempt survivors, suicide loss survivors, and those who have experienced a suicidal crisis can help others understand the complexities of STB, foster empathy through sharing, and generate hope for people at risk. However, lived experience perspectives have historically not been shared broadly, and this is to the detriment of the field's understanding of how best to prevent suicide and provide treatment to those most impacted.

According to the National Strategy for Suicide Prevention (2012) and the Surgeon General's Call to Action on Suicide Prevention (2021), lived experience should be highly valued in the creation and delivery of mental health care. Such perspectives add credibility and value to suicide prevention efforts by going beyond research and academic theory by ensuring that those most impacted by practices and policies are able to contribute to their creation and evaluation. Opportunities to incorporate individuals with lived experience include, but are not limited to, development of care pathways, peer support specialist roles, organizational messaging

R. Willis-Powell (✉)
On Our Own of Maryland, Inc., Elkridge, MD, USA
e-mail: rowan@onourownmd.org

A. Fox
Community Crisis Services, Inc., Hyattsville, MD, USA
e-mail: afox@eastern.edu

J. Cerel
University of Kentucky, College of Social Work, Lexington, KY, USA
e-mail: julie.cerel@uky.edu

© The Author(s) 2022
J. P. Ackerman, L. M. Horowitz (eds.), *Youth Suicide Prevention and Intervention*, SpringerBriefs in Psychology,
https://doi.org/10.1007/978-3-031-06127-1_18

efforts, program evaluation, or meaningful roles on advisory boards for youth suicide prevention efforts. Quality improvement efforts such as a recent PCORI convening grant "Convening Lived Experience & Research Communities to Improve Patient-Centered Outcomes," which brought together individuals with lived experience and suicide prevention researchers to discuss how to integrate lived experience into the design, dissemination, and implementation of research, may be a model for engagement. Lived experience perspectives are especially important when working within mental health service systems with marginalized populations, such as youth, who are often underestimated for not having enough "life experience" to have insight about their own needs. Suicidal thoughts and behaviors are complex and multi-determined; and as such, approach to prevention and treatment requires insight from those who have experienced it themselves.

An important theme that arises when listening to individuals with lived experience is that an early negative experience with disclosure of STB can greatly interfere with future engagement in treatment. Regrettably, there are many instances in which negative disclosure experiences such as shaming lectures or coercive referrals for hospitalization had a lifelong impact on a young person. The stigma around suicide often prevents communication of helpful information in a way that leads to positive support, and the myth that talking about suicide can put ideas of suicide into someone's head is widely detrimental to suicide prevention efforts.

A critical area that the field of suicide prevention must continue to evaluate is the use of involuntary hospitalization as an undifferentiated response to youth suicidal ideation or behavior. This approach may contribute to physical or psychological harm and undermine the autonomy of those most in need of collaborative care. Although inpatient hospitalization may reduce immediate access to lethal means and decrease the amount of time an individual is left alone, this level of care typically offers limited proactive intervention. Rather, the focus of treatment is often on diagnosis, monitoring, stabilization, and medication management (Abas et al., 2003). Many crisis-oriented units focus on short-term safety goals and medication management while limiting the amount of interaction that patients have with family or peers on that unit. The experience of inpatient hospitalization is a major change from everyday life and can be very stressful, especially for young people who are removed from their typical environment, support structures, and coping skills (Lear & Pepper, 2018). This type of disruption can affect identity development also resulting in internalized stigma (Haynes et al., 2011; Polvere, 2011).

Importantly, hospitalization often fails to decrease risk for suicide and can even increase the likelihood of future hospitalization or suicidal behavior (Knesper, 2010). The days and weeks after hospitalization is a period of particularly high risk for further suicidal behavior and even death by suicide (Crawford, 2004; Knesper, 2010). Although deferring to hospitalization when STB is identified is frequently based in good intentions, most patients expressing suicidal ideation are not at imminent risk (Roaten et al., 2021). Disproportionate responses may contribute to devastating negative effects on youth and young adults.

We acknowledge that this chapter departs from traditional academic endeavors by centering on personal lived experience before providing recommendations.

Specifically, we highlight the lived experience of two of the authors during adolescence, with an emphasis on the disclosure of suicidal ideation while centering the importance of lived experience. We then offer insights to drive improved care in acute settings. Utilizing lived experience can help create supportive care environments that are patient-centered, recovery-oriented, and value-driven. To do this effectively, it is important to ask for input and guidance from people with lived experience. We conclude by arguing that when lived experience is valued by the service system, people with mental health diagnoses will face less stigma and experience more compassion when interacting with providers. Given the negative effects of inappropriate provider responses, it is crucial to incorporate insight from those with lived experience to identify the most effective and appropriate care options.

Lived Experiences

Rowan's Lived Experience

When I was 16 years old, I felt like a relatively normal child, yet for a while I had been struggling with post-traumatic stress disorder (PTSD) in response to events occurring in the context of unhealthy relationships. I went in to visit my primary physician for a regular checkup. During that visit, I built up the nerve to disclose to her that I was thinking about killing myself. I let her know that I had experienced thoughts of suicide for a long time but that I did not have a plan or desire to act on my thoughts. It had taken a great deal of courage for me to share this, and unfortunately the result was an immediate referral to the hospital. I felt betrayed and powerless. This traumatic experience contributed to an intense distrust of talking about my passive suicidal ideation even though such thoughts remain present to this day. At the time, my provider asked me a few simple questions, but never asked about the intensity or quality of my suicidal ideation, or even if I had a plan or method to end my life. It did not make sense to me that the person I had reached out to for help encouraged such a restrictive level of care when I was not feeling unsafe. With some luck and fortunate connections, I was able to avoid a 72-h hold at a hospital that night. Because my mother is a social worker, she was able to find me an urgent therapy appointment for the next day. My family's advocacy was the primary reason that I was provided with other options of care that allowed me to avoid additional trauma and financial burden. In retrospect, I can understand that my provider was probably scared, uncomfortable, and unsure of what to do, and although she was concerned with my safety, she likely had no other tools except hospitalization when confronted with a teen with thoughts of suicide. I have witnessed this fear and discomfort in many providers with whom I have interacted over the years as a patient and as a professional. It is a fear that I understand deeply as a passionate youth advocate and as someone with a younger sibling who struggles with suicidal thoughts. But in my advocacy work, I have seen the harm that can be done when the care provided is based on fear. Examples are when fear of liability comes before patient well-being and when providers lack specific training in managing suicide risk through care pathways that are informed by lived experience perspectives.

My provider's overreaction has stuck with me to this day. Providers should be aware that how they respond to youth in crisis contributes to whether they seek help in the future. I rarely bring up suicidal ideation with anyone now, and when I do, I sanitize my descriptions and make sure I label it as "passive" due to a fear of being hospitalized. If my provider had been trained to explore my suicidal ideation with empathy rather than fear and discussed the range of options available for me, then the result would not likely have been hospitalization to meet my needs. Rather, establishing a collaborative plan for safety would have been the priority and led to a better outcome. I would also feel more comfortable disclosing suicidal ideation to providers now.

In my work as a mentor and advocate for young adults with lived experience in Maryland, I frequently tell the youth with whom I work to be specific when they describe their suicidal ideation to their providers, and to be ready to advocate for what they want their care to look like, so they are not hospitalized without a clear justification. My job is to mentor and support young adults with lived experience who have an interest in advocacy and peer support, and that includes teaching them how to advocate for themselves and their recovery needs.

Amanda's Lived Experience

As I entered my teenage years, I began struggling with mental illness, including thoughts of suicide. My family didn't know anything about mental health care or how to get me help. I already felt like a burden and wanted to protect them, so I hid as much from them as possible. My depression worsened and when I was about 15, I had my first suicide attempt. When my mom took me to my primary care doctor after this attempt, my doctor lectured me about why I should want to live. I was struggling intensely, and instead of having a conversation about the pain that led me to seek to end my life, I was shamed for my act of desperation. My doctor told my mom that "I would be fine because I had vomited" and told her to take me home without additional precautions. I had to research my own mental health needs and treatment options. Then I had to personally educate my parents in order to get any type of mental health treatment.

When I was later admitted for inpatient hospitalization years later for a separate suicide attempt, I was horrified at the way people who were struggling to manage severe distress were treated by hospital staff. It was like those admitted had lost the right to be treated like a human simply for experiencing an emotional crisis. Personally, inpatient care has been minimally therapeutic, and really only ensured that I did not have access to things to harm myself with (even this was not effective). I have been on different types of psychiatric units and have found that more special-ized units tend to offer higher-quality suicide-specific care. Nevertheless, the most helpful part of treatment for me has been the shared experiences and friends that I have met along the way. The support and comradery that develops between people who truly understand what it is like to live through these struggles is empowering. Other things that have been helpful for me are connecting with clinicians who understand the process of level of care assessments and proper safety planning, which have allowed me to stay safe without being admitted to an inpatient unit for years since these initial distressing experiences.

Other Learning Experiences

In our advocacy roles, we have learned that many youth face unhelpful reactions when first disclosing their experiences of suicidal thoughts to adults who are under-prepared to respond effectively. Specifically, we have heard responses ranging from a young elementary student being told by their parents that they are "just overreact-ing" and "can't possibly have feelings of wanting to die" to a 16-year-old being hospitalized without so much as a conversation.

Yet, we have also witnessed providers discuss suicidal ideation and past attempts in a curious and empathetic way which typically leads to better outcomes for young people. In one instance, a young woman screened positive for suicide risk at a pri-mary care visit. Instead of immediate hospitalization, the provider conducted a brief suicide safety assessment and a collaborative safety plan. Her provider asked her multiple questions about what her suicidal ideation looked like, how it was impact-ing her, whether it was passive or active, and if she had a plan to end her life. Based on the safety assessment and commitment to her safety plan, the provider and patient together agreed that hospitalization was not necessary because the patient was not expressing active suicidal ideation and was not at imminent risk for suicide. The provider conducted a follow-up call with the patient. As a result, this young woman spoke highly of her interactions with providers and had a positive outlook on services available to help her through a suicidal crisis. The clinician's process emphasized the patient's agency in decision-making and safety planning. This posi-tive experience set her up to be able to disclose suicidal ideation to providers in the future because she felt the provider would conduct further assessment to determine the appropriate disposition.

Discussion

The lived experience of struggling with suicidal ideation and having difficult con-versations of disclosure, as detailed in our stories above, have shaped our views of what kind of supports are helpful versus harmful. We recognize that unhelpful pro-vider reactions are primarily caused by two things: (1) a lack of training on suicide-specific screening, assessment, and treatment for providers and (2) a tendency for providers to respond from a place of fear/discomfort. That fear may be due to discomfort managing suicide risk, liability concerns (e.g., fear of being sued if a client dies by suicide), or misconceptions about the best ways to protect children. Most mental health clinicians feel that they have not been appropriately trained to adequately help suicidal youth (Schmitz et al., 2012). There are important lessons to learn from these anecdotes above that unfortunately are common among youth with suicidal ideation. To address these issues, we present recommendations for providers.

Recommendations for Discussing Suicide

As people with lived experiences, we make three recommendations for clinicians who encounter patients with suicidal ideation: (1) First, clinicians should do an internal assessment about what they feel about youth with suicidal thoughts so they can understand their personal biases and make sure they respond to young people who are struggling with compassion and without judgment. (2) Second, clinicians should listen to and fully discuss with patients what suicidal ideation means to the patient, ask about personal triggers and warning signs, and ask specifically what suicidal thoughts and behaviors look like for that person. (3) Lastly, they should provide options other than hospitalization taking into account the patient's support system and a willingness to contribute collaboratively to safety decisions.

The use of safety plans with suicidal youth is critical (see Monahan & Stanley, Chap. 9, this volume) so that nuanced decisions around safety and level of care recommendations can be made without unnecessarily restrictive hospitalizations. In our own lives and our work, we have witnessed a lack of options presented to youth and their families. We have seen youth hospitalized multiple times in a single year due to a lack of alternatives presented to the family, and we believe that the patient should not have to be an expert in mental health treatment systems in order to receive appropriate care, nor should they need special connections to guarantee appropriate supports. It is important for families to know that there are other options other than hospitalization which could better suit their needs. Intensive outpatient (IOP) programs, crisis counseling, an emergency therapy appointment, or peer support providers are examples of appealing alternatives.

Many communities are taking meaningful steps to reduce the frequency of hospitalizations among youth. One key approach is an increase in peer support specialists working in wellness and recovery centers, emergency rooms, and mobile crisis teams. Individuals in these roles are often adept at de-escalating someone in crisis and have connections and knowledge about the available services in the area. They are trained to take the time to sit with a youth who is in crisis and talk with them about the options available, which often allows the youth to find an option that is a better fit for their needs.

Additionally, evidence-based treatments are available that decrease the need for emergency department visits. We have seen hospital units who staff peer supporters and engage patients in creating a Wellness Recovery Action Plan (WRAP) and are committed to making what can be a traumatic experience more recovery oriented. Providers should prioritize safety planning while educating youth and families about different treatment options that extend beyond crisis care and medication management. Patients prefer to be informed of treatment options (Bellairs-Walsh et al., 2020), and safety planning may increase perceptions of agency.

Training providers to have empathic nonjudgmental conversations with young people and improving comfort level in working with people who have thoughts of suicide is critical. A recent study found that individuals weigh the costs and benefits associated with disclosure of suicidal ideation and only disclose when the perceived benefits outweigh the perceived costs (Frey et al., 2018). They are most likely to disclose to a confidant, a person who has responded compassionately to disclosures of suicidal ideation previously, or someone who had known about past suicidal behavior and been emotionally supportive. Unfortunately, our experiences and existing research suggest that many providers have inadequate training for detecting and managing suicide risk. Many clinicians, especially those with limited experience, are unable to accurately determine when hospitalization is the best choice (Stulz et al., 2015). One reason for this is that few states require clinicians to receive formal training in suicide risk assessment and safety planning. For providers, suicide-specific treatments like the Collaborative Assessment and Management of Suicidality (CAMS; Gould et al., 2013; Jobes, 2012; Smith-Osbourne et al., 2017) or Lifeworks' ASIST: Applied Suicide Intervention Skills Training (Ashwood et al., 2015) may guide how to interact with a suicidal person.

Conclusions

Each of these recommendations requires a culture shift within healthcare systems and will require increased research and funding to meet the increased need for suicide prevention and treatment services in the USA. From our work, we know responding to suicidal ideation is an incredibly complex task that can have a significant emotional impact. Youth experiencing suicidal ideation should feel supported and empowered in the care they receive. We ask that providers enter into conversations about suicidal ideation with the intent to listen and ask questions, engage the youth in the process of safety planning, provide alternatives to hospitalization whenever safe to do so, and collaboratively decide how to stay alive.

References

Abas, M., Vanderpyl, J., Le Prou, T., Kydd, R., Emery, B., & Foliaki, S. A. (2003). Psychiatric hospitalization: Reasons for admission and alternatives to admission in South Auckland, New Zealand. *The Australian and New Zealand Journal of Psychiatry, 37*(5), 620–625. https://doi.org/10.1046/j.1440-1614.2003.01229.x

Ashwood, J. S., Briscombe, B., Ramchand, R., May, E., & Burnam, M. A. (2015). Analysis of the benefits and costs of CalMHSA's investment in Applied Suicide Intervention Skills Training (ASIST). *Rand Health Quarterly, 5*(2), 9.

Bellairs-Walsh, I., Perry, Y., Krysinska, K., Byrne, S. J., Boland, A., Michail, M., Lamblin, M., Gibson, K. L., Lin, A., Li, T. Y., Hetrick, S., & Robinson, J. (2020). Best practice when working with suicidal behaviour and self-harm in primary care: a qualitative exploration of young people's perspectives. *BMJ open, 10(10), e038855.* https://doi.org/10.1136/bmjopen-2020-038855

Crawford, M. J. (2004). Suicide following discharge from in-patient psychiatric care. *Advances in Psychiatric Treatment, 10*(6), 434–438. https://doi.org/10.1192/apt.10.6.434

Frey, L. M., Fulginiti, A., Lezine, D., & Cerel, J. (2018). The decision-making process for disclosing suicidal ideation and behavior to family and friends. *Family Relations, 67*(3), 414–427. https://doi.org/10.1111/fare.12315

Gould, M. S., Cross, W., Pisani, A. R., Munfakh, J. L., & Kleinman, M. (2013). Impact of applied suicide intervention skills training on the national suicide prevention lifeline. *Suicide & Life-Threatening Behavior, 43*(6), 676–691. https://doi.org/10.1111/sltb.12049

Haynes, C., Eivors, A., & Crossley, J. (2011). 'Living in an alternative reality': Adolescents' experiences of psychiatric inpatient care. *Child and Adolescent Mental Health, 16*(3), 150–157. https://doi.org/10.1111/j.1475-3588.2011.00598.x

Jobes, D. A. (2012). The Collaborative Assessment and Management of Suicidality (CAMS): An evolving evidence-based clinical approach to suicidal risk. *Suicide & Life-Threatening Behavior, 42*(6), 640–653. https://doi.org/10.1111/j.1943-278X.2012.00119.x

Knesper, D. J. (2010). *Continuity of care for suicide prevention and research: Suicide attempts and suicide deaths subsequent to discharge from the emergency department or psychiatry inpatient unit.* Suicide Prevention Resource Center.

Lear, M. K., & Pepper, C. M. (2018). Family-based outpatient treatments: A viable alternative to hospitalization for suicidal adolescents. *Journal of Family Therapy, 40*(1), 83–99. https://doi.org/10.1111/1467-6427.12146

Polvere, L. (2011). Youth Perspectives on Restrictive Mental Health Placement: Unearthing a Counter Narrative. *Journal of Adolescent Research, 26(3), 318–343.* https://doi.org/10.1177/0743558410391257

Roaten, K., Horowitz, L. M., Bridge, J. A., Goans, C., McKintosh, C., Genzel, R., Johnson, C., & North, C. S. (2021). Universal pediatric suicide risk screening in a health care system: 90,000 patient encounters. *Journal of the Academy of Consultation-Liaison Psychiatry, 62*(4), 421–429. https://doi.org/10.1016/j.jaclp.2020.12.002

Schmitz, W. M., Allen, M. H., Feldman, B. N., Gutin, N. J., Jahn, D. R., Kleespies, P. M., Quinnett, P., & Simpson, S. (2012). Preventing suicide through improved training in suicide assessment and care: An American Association of Suicidology Task Force report addressing serious gaps in U.S. mental health training. *Suicide and Life-threatening Behavior, 42*(3), 292–304. https://doi.org/10.1111/j.1943-278X.2012.00090.x

Smith-Osborne, A., Maleku, A., & Morgan, S. (2017). Impact of applied suicide intervention skills training on resilience and suicide risk in army reserve units. *Traumatology, 23*(1), 49. https://doi.org/10.1037/trm0000092

Stulz, N., Nevely, A., Hilpert, M., Bielinski, D., Spisla, C., Maeck, L., & Hepp, U. (2015). Referral to inpatient treatment does not necessarily imply a need for inpatient treatment. *Administration and Policy in Mental Health, 42*(4), 474–483. https://doi.org/10.1007/s10488-014-0561-5

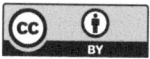

The manufacturer's authorised representative in the EU is Springer
Nature Customer Service Centre GmbH, Europaplatz 3, 69115 Heidelberg,
Germany. If you have any concerns regarding our products, please
contact ProductSafety@springernature.com

Printed and bound by CPI Group (UK) Ltd, Croydon, CR0 4YY
29/04/2026
02099459-0019